ARTIFICIAL INTELLIGENCE IN SPORT PERFORMANCE ANALYSIS

To understand the dynamic patterns of behaviours and interactions between athletes that characterize successful performance in different sports is an important challenge for all sport practitioners. This book guides the reader in understanding how an ecological dynamics framework for use of artificial intelligence (AI) can be implemented to interpret sport performance and the design of practice contexts.

By examining how AI methodologies are utilized in team games, such as football, as well as in individual sports, such as golf and climbing, this book provides a better understanding of the kinematic and physiological indicators that might better capture athletic performance by looking at the current state-of-the-art AI approaches.

Artificial Intelligence in Sport Performance Analysis provides an all-encompassing perspective in an innovative approach that signals practical applications for both academics and practitioners in the fields of coaching, sports analysis, and sport science, as well as related subjects such as engineering, computer and data science, and statistics.

Duarte Araújo is Associate Professor and Head of CIPER – Interdisciplinary Centre for the Study of Human Performance – and Director of the Laboratory of Expertise in Sport of the Faculty of Human Kinetics at the University of Lisbon, Portugal.

Micael Couceiro is Associate Researcher at the Institute of Systems and Robotics, Coimbra, Portugal. He is also co-founder and CEO of the company Ingeniarius.

Ludovic Seifert is Professor of Motor Control and Learning, Deputy Dean of the CETAPS Lab, and Head of the Sport Performance Analysis and Big Data Master's degree at the Faculty of Sport Sciences, University of Rouen Normandie, France.

Hugo Sarmento is Assistant Professor in the Faculty of Sport Sciences and Physical Education, University of Coimbra, Portugal.

Keith Davids is Professor of Motor Learning in the Sport and Human Performance research group, Sheffield Hallam University, UK.

ARTIFICIAL INTELLIGENCE IN SPORT PERFORMANCE ANALYSIS

Duarte Araújo, Micael Couceiro, Ludovic Seifert, Hugo Sarmento, and Keith Davids

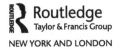
Routledge
Taylor & Francis Group

NEW YORK AND LONDON

First published 2021
by Routledge
52 Vanderbilt Avenue, New York, NY 10017

and by Routledge
2 Park Square, Milton Park, Abingdon, Oxon, OX14 4RN

Routledge is an imprint of the Taylor & Francis Group, an informa business

Library of Congress Cataloging-in-Publication Data
Names: Araújo, Duarte, author. | Couceiro, Micael, author. |
Seifert, Ludovic, author. | Sarmento, Hugo, author. |
Davids, K. (Keith), 1953– author.
Title: Artificial intelligence in sport performance analysis /
Duarte Araújo, Micael Couceiro, Ludovic Seifert, Hugo Sarmento,
and Keith Davids.
Description: New York : Routledge, 2020. | Includes bibliographical
references and index.
Identifiers: LCCN 2020050451 (print) | LCCN 2020050452
(ebook) | ISBN 9780367254360 (Hardback) | ISBN 9780367254377
(Paperback) | ISBN 9781003163589 (eBook)
Subjects: LCSH: Sports—Physiological aspects. | Artificial
intelligence. | Sports—Physiological aspects—Research—
Methodology. | Performance—Data processing. | Sports sciences—
Data processing. | Performance—Research—Methodology.
Classification: LCC RC1235 .A73 2020 (print) | LCC RC1235
(ebook) | DDC 612/.0440285—dc23
LC record available at https://lccn.loc.gov/2020050451
LC ebook record available at https://lccn.loc.gov/2020050452

ISBN: 978-0-367-25436-0 (hbk)
ISBN: 978-0-367-25437-7 (pbk)
ISBN: 978-1-003-16358-9 (ebk)

Typeset in Bembo
by codeMantra

CONTENTS

FIGURES

TABLES

AUTHORS

Duarte Araújo, Ph.D., is Associate Professor and Head of the Department of Sport and Health and Faculty of Human Kinetics at the University of Lisbon, Portugal. He leads both the research centre of this school, CIPER, and the Laboratory of Expertise in Sport. He is an associate editor of the journal *Psychology of Sport and Exercise* as well as the *Journal of Expertise*. Araújo's research on sport expertise and decision-making, performance analysis, and affordances for physical activity has been funded by the Fundação para a Ciência e a Tecnologia. He has published more than 160 papers in scientific journals (with over 5,500 citations in the Web of Science) and more than 15 books about expertise, team performance, variability, cognition, and decision-making in sport. He collaborates regularly with Sport Federations and Clubs and supervises several doctoral students from Portugal, Italy, Brazil, Spain, and Australia.

Micael Couceiro obtained the B.Sc., Teaching Licensure, and M.Sc. degrees in Electrical Engineering from the Engineering Institute of Coimbra, and the Ph.D. degree in Electrical and Computer Engineering from the University of Coimbra. He completed the postdoc studies on Human Kinetics at the Faculty of Human Kinetics of the University of Lisbon. Over the past 14 years, he has been conducting scientific research on several areas, including robotics, computer vision, sports engineering, and others. This resulted in more than 50 articles in international impact factor journals, more than 70 articles at international conferences, three books, 15 M.Sc. students' supervision, two ongoing Ph.D. students' supervision, and the coordination of six R&D projects. He is currently an Associate Researcher at the Institute of Systems and Robotics. He is also the co-founder and CEO of Ingeniarius – a company devoted to the development of robotic solutions and wearable technologies.

Keith Davids, Ph.D., is a professor of motor learning at the Sport & Human Performance Research Group in Sheffield Hallam University, UK. He graduated from the University of London and obtained a Ph.D. in psychology and physical education from the University of Leeds. He has previously held professorial positions in the United Kingdom (Manchester Metropolitan University), New Zealand (University of Otago), Australia (Queensland University of Technology), and Finland (Finnish Distinguished Professor in the faculty of sport and health sciences at the University of Jyväskylä). Davids' research programme investigates sport performance, skill acquisition, and expertise enhancement in sport and how to design learning, training, and practice environments to successfully achieve these outcomes. He collaborates on research in sport, physical activity, and exercise with colleagues at universities in Spain, Portugal, France, the Netherlands, Iran, Macedonia, New Zealand, Australia, and Finland. A large proportion of his scientific and practical research has been undertaken in collaboration with the New Zealand South Island Sports Academy, the Queensland Academy of Sport, the Australian Institute of Sport, Diving Australia, Cricket Australia, GB Cycling, and the English Institute of Sport.

Hugo Sarmento, Ph.D., is an assistant professor at the University of Coimbra, Portugal. He is the head of the master's programme in Youth Sport Training. Sarmento's research is on sport expertise and talent development following an ecological dynamics approach. He has also conducted studies in performance analysis, training load monitoring, match analysis, small-sided and conditioned games, and physical activity and health. He has published more than 80 international peer-reviewed original articles. Additionally, he is a member of six editorial boards of international scientific journals.

Ludovic Seifert, Ph.D., is a professor at the University of Rouen Normandy, France. He is the vice dean of the Centre d'Etudes des Transformations des Activités Physiques et Sportives (CETAPS) lab and the head of the master's programme in sport performance analysis. He obtained a certificate in physical education in 1998 and a Ph.D. degree in sport science from the University of Rouen Normandy in 2003. Seifert's field of research relates to motor control and learning and expertise and talent development following an ecological dynamics approach. His emphasis focuses on movement coordination and visual motor skills, with a particular interest in swimming and climbing. Such topics have led him to work closely with several French sport federations (such as swimming, climbing and mountaineering, and ice hockey) and professional clubs. His research has been published and cited extensively in peer-reviewed journals.

PREFACE

Technology in general, and digital computers in particular, has had a profound impact on sport. Practitioners rely on digital data to monitor and enhance performance. Officials use tracking systems to augment their judgement. Audiences use collective shared data purported to expand the places in which sports can be watched and experienced. Extracting big data from the dynamics of sport performance is becoming a regular procedure in major sport events.

Currently, an important challenge for sport practitioners and scientists is to understand the dynamic patterns of behaviour and interaction among athletes that characterize successful performance in different sports. For this, the use of artificial intelligence (AI) methodologies is becoming increasingly popular. AI research has created and developed hardware and software systems that can record, classify, analyse, and interpret large amounts of data. However, one risk of AI research is to be data-driven. This textbook advances the argument that data-informed decision-making is needed to engage learners, coaches, and performers, instead of data-driven approaches. This requires a comprehensive theoretical framework to critically interpret the information from the large and complex datasets for enhancing athlete performance in training and competition. This textbook proposes an ecological dynamics framework to guide the reader in understanding how to use AI methodologies in sport performance analysis. The book adopts team sports, in particular football, as task vehicles, while additionally focusing on how AI methodologies are utilized in individual sports, such as golf, swimming, and climbing, among others.

Part of the power of big data comes from the potential for using AI, in particular machine learning, to identify coherent patterns in the data. Importantly, human observers are needed in these processes to monitor automatically created results to determine which patterns are meaningful and which are random

(Woo, Tay, & Proctor, 2020). AI methods have the goal of creating reliable and replicable prediction models from datasets that may have a large number of different variables. To handle the large number of variables efficiently, these algorithms can be used to search the predictor space and highlight variables with explanatory power. The methods do not guarantee that an ideal model is found, but instead they can find a model that performs well under a variety of conditions, offering better diagnostics and interventions.

The main objective of the book is to provide guidelines for research and practice in sport performance analysis, including the following:

a   To provide a better understanding of the kinematic and physiological indicators that might better capture performance, namely when capturing the performer-environment system in ecophysical variables, by looking at the current state of the art;

b   To delineate research designs, focusing on participants, tasks, contexts, and procedures, as well as the necessary data acquisition technology;

c   To identify computational metrics that support interpretation of spatio-temporal variables underpinning athlete performance while, at the same time, functioning as data pre-processing routines to extract representative features of competitive performance.

d   To provide an understanding of athletic performance by automatically assessing athletes' behaviours and, to some extent, predicting health and performance outcomes, using AI approaches.

Artificial Intelligence in Sport Performance Analysis provides an all-encompassing perspective in an innovative approach that signals practical applications for coaches, sports analysts, sport scientists, and practitioners, through condensing a large volume of data into a smaller set of variables, and providing a deeper analysis than available in typical measures of performance outcomes of competitive sports. It explains how dynamic patterns of data can be interpreted and used by sport practitioners to understand successful and less successful performance behaviours, and guide performance preparation and the design of training and practice contexts.

This book contains seven chapters. Chapters 1 and 2 provide an overview of the concepts and research, focusing on big data and artificial intelligence in sports. Chapter 1 discusses how to deal with Big Data. This discussion provides a summary of recent approaches adopted to improve the interpretation of large and complex volumes of data in order to avoid falling back into the mere datafication of sports, thus leading from traditional methods for quantifying sport performances to a pattern-driven quantification further described in Chapter 2. In Chapter 2, a state-of-the-art review is presented clarifying how competition results, scoring, and injuries occurrences have been explored by means of artificial intelligence. Next, Chapter 3 presents a guide for setting up research designs in sports. This chapter highlights variables that describe sport performance by centring its discussion on kinematic and physiological performance indicators, and how to move from them to ecophysical variables. It examines the application of these 'low level' performance indicators in sports, such as football, describing various methods that have been used to investigate the demands of sports. It describes the representativeness of accurate and reliable time-motion kinematical analysis, such as the position of players in the field or their body pose, so as to provide a more comprehensive understanding of the performance. Chapter 3 also highlights the use of automated tools for assisting the behavioural analysis of performance in sports to make the difference in improving the individual and collective outcomes. It explains how to prepare and build the methodological setup to analyse athletic performance. Several methodological and technological alternatives are presented and compared, such as traditional cameras, 3D depth cameras, motion capture suits, and sport-specific devices, supporting the design in both research and practice. The aim of Chapter 4 is to move from the extracted variables to processing representative features of the spatiotemporal variables characterizing performance of performers, presenting the most up-to-date methods and measures adopted in football, as a primary case study. Chapters 5 and 6 revolve around the use of artificial intelligence to recognize patterns in sport performance, presenting classification architectures designed to classify and, to some extent, predict athlete's health and performance outcomes. The book concludes by summarizing the main contributions, identifying key messages for readers, delineating some limitations inherent to several approaches that are introduced, suggesting future directions for readers, and presenting implications of artificial intelligence for research, education, and training contexts.

The book is aimed at those delivering and taking undergraduate and postgraduate modules in sport sciences, performance analysis, and related areas. It is also relevant for practitioners working in sports organizations seeking to implement new technologies and AI procedures to enhance understanding of dynamics patterns of interactions in sports. The topic of this book captures the attention of coaches, performance analysts, sport engineers, and sport scientists working in the industry and in professional sport clubs.

An important difference for this book is that it follows an ecological dynamics theoretical framework. For present purposes, we highlight three of the key theoretical assumptions that integrate the many facets of the ecological dynamics framework (Araújo et al., 2020; Button et al., 2020): (1) performance emerges from the performer-environment system; (2) to understand the performance of an individual, an analysis of the behaviours offered by his/her environment (i.e., affordances or opportunities for action) is necessary; and (3) performance emerges (as a result of self-organization) under interacting constraints for in-depth descriptions of the ecological dynamics approach to sport performance.

First, performer and environment function relationally rather than independently. Performers act intentionally immersed in a wide range of circumstantial factors that are typically changing. Since athletes are participants in a complex dynamic system, each person's action continually must be re-adjusted with respect to changing circumstances. Also, what defines the performer-environment system at any moment is not fixed, but continually shifts as the focus of a performer's action changes. This indicates that action is not just limited to processes occurring only in the person (i.e., physiological or mental). Contrary to this organismic-centred tendency, for the ecological dynamics approach, behaviour is a reorganization of the organism-environment system. The implication of this idea is that performance can only be understood not simply according to the characteristics of a performer, but symmetrically according to the characteristics of a performance environment.

Second, for a performer, the environment is experienced as being meaningful, implying that an understanding of performance should embed experiences in environmental properties, as Gibson (1979) theorized with his concept of affordances. Environmental properties can directly inform an individual performer about what he/she can and cannot do in a performance environment. An affordance is a property of the environment taken with reference to the capabilities of a performer. Consequently, it is understandable that perceiving is a process of detecting information for specific action possibilities in the environment.

Third, considering the performer-environment system, performance can be understood as self-organized under constraints, in contrast to the organization being imposed from inside (e.g., the mind) or outside (e.g., coach's instructions). Performance is not prescribed by internal or external structures, yet within existing constraints, there are typically a limited number of stable solutions that can achieve specific desired outcomes. When a system (i.e., the performer-environment system) establishes a state (i.e., behaviour pattern) only because of the dynamical interactions among individual components within the system, the state is self-organized. External processes (e.g., coach's plan) do not cause self-organization; rather, this process is generated by components within the system (e.g., player, teammates, adversaries, coach and technical staff, facilities). Behaviour patterns that emerge are different from the components that make up the system, and cannot be predicted solely from the characteristics of the individual components.

Ecological dynamics implies that ecophysical variables (Araújo et al., 2020) provide the most appropriate starting point to capture intelligent behaviour. These are variables that express the fit between the environment and the performer's adaptations. Anyway, the interpretation of such variables may benefit from the expertise of sport practitioners. Thus, visual analytics is highly encouraged as a tool for interpreting big data, where its display can be developed in an interdisciplinary way, with the contribution of sport scientists and practitioners, computer and data scientists, and engineers (Couceiro et al., 2016). Visual analytics and carefully developed infographics may be well placed to consider the context, in a way that an automated, context-free output may never offer. Given the expertise of sport scientists to understand how movement, body, and context contributes to understand intelligent performance behaviours, they can work together with computer scientists in developing less mentalist, and more embodied and embedded, architectures for capturing the impact of artificial intelligence. This is the main aim of this book.

31 October 2020

Duarte Araújo; Micael Couceiro, Ludovic Seifert,

Hugo Sarmento, and Keith Davids

REFERENCES

Araújo, D., Davids, K., & Renshaw, I. (2020). Cognition, emotion and action in sport: An ecological dynamics perspective. In G. Tenenbaum & R. Eklund (Eds.), *Handbook of sport psychology* (4th ed., pp. 535–555). New York, NY: John Wiley & Sons, Inc.

Button, C., Seifert, L., Chow, J. Y., Araújo, D., & Davids, K. (2020). *Dynamics of skill acquisition: An ecological dynamics approach* (2nd ed.). Champaign, IL: Human Kinetics.

Couceiro, M. S., Dias, G., Araújo, D., & Davids, K. (2016). The ARCANE project: How an ecological dynamics framework can enhance performance assessment and prediction in football. *Sports Medicine, 46*(12), 1781–1786.

Gibson, J. J. (1979). *The ecological approach to visual perception*. Boston, MA: Houghton Mifflin.

Woo, S. E., Tay, L., & Proctor, R. W. (Eds.). (2020). *Big data in psychological research*. Washington, DC: American Psychological Association.

ACKNOWLEDGEMENTS

Duarte Araújo's work was supported by Portuguese Science Agency 'Fundação para a Ciência e Tecnologia' under grant number UIDB/00447/2020 attributed to CIPER – Centro Interdisciplinar para o Estudo da Performance Humana (unit 447).

Micael Couceiro's work was supported by the CORE R&D Project, which was cofunded by the Portugal 2020 programme, under the reference CENTRO-01-0247-FEDER 037082. For more details visit http://core.ingeniarius.pt/.

Ludovic Seifert's work was supported by the French National Agency of Research under DynACEV grant (ID: ANR-17-CE38-0006) and NePTUNE grant (ID: ANR-19-STHP-0004).

1

EMPOWERING HUMAN INTELLIGENCE

The Ecological Dynamics Approach to Big Data and Artificial Intelligence in Sport Performance Preparation

Big Data in Sport

Digital technology has had a profound impact on sport (Miah, 2017). Athletes and coaches rely on digital data to monitor and enhance the performance. Officials use tracking systems to augment their judgement. Audiences use collective shared data purported to expand the places in which sports can be watched and experienced.

Nowadays, technology enables practitioners, performers, and spectators to collect and store a massive amount of data in faster, more abundant, and more diverse ways than ever. Data can be collected from various sensors and devices in different formats, from independent or connected applications. This data avalanche has outpaced human capability to process, analyse, store, and understand the information contained in these datasets. Moreover, people and devices are becoming increasingly interconnected. The increase in the number of such connected components generates a massive dataset, and valuable information needs to be discovered from patterns within the data to help improve performance, safety, health, and well-being. Not only have technological advancements led to an abundance of new data streams, repositories, and computational power, but they also have resulted in advances in statistical and computational techniques, such as artificial intelligence, that have proliferated widespread analysis of such datasets in many domains, including sport, improving our ability to plan, prepare, and predict performance outcomes. Therefore, it is unsurprising that big data is also entering research programmes in the sport sciences (Goes et al., 2020; Rein & Memmert, 2016; Chapter 2). Big data broadly refers to multiplying multiform data (e.g., structured, unstructured) and their supporting technological infrastructure (i.e., capture, storage, processing) and analytic techniques that can enhance research (Woo, Tay, & Proctor, 2020).

Big data, a term probably coined by John Mashey in the mid-1990s (Gandomi & Haider, 2015), is used to identify datasets that cannot be managed for a particular problem domain with traditional methodologies to obtain meaning, due to their large size and complexity (Proctor & Xiong, 2020). Consequently, Volume, Variety, and Velocity (the three Vs) have emerged as a common framework to describe big data. It is relevant to understand the meaning of the three Vs (Gandomi & Haider, 2015): (i) Volume is related to the size of data (many terabytes and even exabytes); (ii) Variety refers to the types of data (e.g., text, physical sensors data, audio, video, graph) and its structure (e.g., structured or unstructured); (iii) Velocity indicates the continuous generation of streams of data and the speed at which those data should be analysed. There are additional Vs being discussed nowadays (Proctor & Xiong, 2020) such as Variability (variation in the data flow), Veracity (imprecision of the data), and Value (obtain meaning to inform decisions in ways only possible with big data). Relatedly, big data mining is the capability of obtaining useful information from these large datasets (Fan & Bifet, 2014). One way of mining big data is by means of artificial intelligence, as described in the remaining chapters of this book.

For sport scientists and practitioners, the challenges start from understanding how to obtain and access data, followed by how to process and clean big data into formats usable for research and athlete support goals (Endel & Piringer, 2015). At the same time, the collected data may be incomplete, which requires methods to transform, detect, and deal with missing data. Also, the traditional statistical method of null hypothesis testing at 0.05 alpha level loses its meaning because very small differences can be statistically significant due to the very large sample sizes involved in big datasets. Thus, one obvious accompanying challenge is to understand how to obtain meaningful information and predictions from big data. One solution is to place more emphasis on statistics and computational modelling (Proctor & Xiong, 2020), such as machine learning (e.g., Couceiro, Dias, Mendes, & Araújo, 2013, see Chapter 2 for a review). Another possible complementary solution, discussed at the end of this chapter, is to become theoretically informed about what data to obtain, how to process it, and how to interpret it, instead of simply relying on computational brute force.

Sources of Big Data

Woo, Tay, Jebb, Ford, and Kern (2020) identified three major sources of big data as most frequently mentioned or used in current behavioural research: social media (e.g., Twitter, Facebook), wearable sensors (e.g., Garmin, Fitbit), and Internet activities (e.g., Internet searches, page views). Woo, Tay, Jebb, and colleagues (2020) also identified two other emergent data sources that provide an increasing amount of accessible data: public network cameras and smartphones (see Chapter 3 for the main sources used in sport sciences). These big data sources are different from more 'traditional' data sources (e.g., surveys, interviews) because the latter are typically much smaller in size, more slowly generated, and less technological. Importantly, 'small' and 'big' data range on a continuum rather than represent two distinct categories.

Recent advances in such technology have improved the ability to study sport performance (see Chapter 3) and the expression of expertise processes as they naturally occur (e.g., Baker & Farrow, 2015; Ericsson, Hoffman, Kozbelt, & Williams, 2018; Ward, Schraagen, Gore, & Roth, 2020). Ecological momentary assessment (EMA), which collects behavioural moment-by-moment data using electronic handheld devices, requires participants to answer questionnaires several times a day after being prompted by those devices. Although these devices can capture behavioural processes *in situ*, limitations such as survey fatigue, limitations in verbalizing behaviour, and limitations of response bias may influence self-report survey responses of participants (Blake, Lee, Rosa, & Sherman, 2020). Mobile sensing, using smartphones, is a more recent approach to collect data of naturalistic behaviour (e.g., Araújo, Brymer, Brito, Withagen, & Davids, 2019). Mobile sensing unobtrusively tracks a participant's physical location, his/her physical activity, and his/her physiological information (Júdice et al., 2020; Ram & Diehl, 2015). Sensors with Internet connectivity can provide a continuous stream of data. Many types of sensors could be inserted in wearables to collect specific data such as pressure sensors, accelerometers, and positional data (e.g., GIS and GPS, where GIS – stands for Geographical Information System – is a software program that helps people use the information that is collected from the GPS – Global Positioning System – satellites) (Woo, Tay, Jebb, et al., 2020). Each of these sensors can capture variables of physical behaviour, including location, posture, and movement (e.g., sitting, standing, walking, running), and physical proximity to other sensors (Chaffin et al., 2017). These technologies are ever-expanding, and can capture types of behavioural data not accessible previously, due to privacy and confidentiality concerns, costs, and practical limitations (Woo, Tay, Jebb, et al., 2020). What may be a unique advantage of smartphones is that they are highly portable, enabling researchers to cross survey data with behavioural (and often social media) observations recorded and shared through smartphone sensors, and plug-ins to capture a holistic account of participants' behaviours and experiences (Harari et al., 2016, but see Fortes et al., 2019). Discussions of reliability and validity of behavioural measurements using smartphone data have been recently offered (Harari et al., 2016; Júdice et al., 2020; Woo, Tay, Jebb, et al., 2020).

Although advances in wearables capture important aspects of a person's environment, they provide no visual sense of what the person has encountered during their actions or how a setting may have visually changed. A wearable camera can provide raw information about an individual's visual environment and can fill this gap in the collection of naturalistic behaviour (Omodei & McLennan, 1994). Another possibility for performances in limited spaces is video recordings of single-person (e.g., golf) or interpersonal interactions such as those between athletes and teams and a performance environment. In the 1980s and 1990s, these video recordings were often coded and summarized; however, recent studies have implemented more intensive data collection strategies to examine group behaviours in sport (Araújo & Davids, 2016; Rein & Memmert, 2016). There are also video data available through public cameras, which usually have insufficient image resolution for fine-grained, individual-level behavioural analyses. However, they can still be used to capture some essential observations and meaningful patterns of individual, interpersonal, and group behaviours in public spaces, such as behaviours (e.g., physical activity) in public locations or crowd behaviours in sport events (Woo, Tay, Jebb et al., 2020). And these methods are rapidly improving to become a valid and useful approach (Adolph, 2016). Moreover, video recordings' metric properties require careful *a priori* decisions on the appropriate unit of analysis for assessing the constructs of interest and boundaries around the time frame and what aspects of the image are included or excluded (e.g., Sanchez-Algarra & Anguera, 2013).

Validity and Reliability of Big Data Measurements

Big data sources include practical and ethical challenges, such as privacy, data security and storage, data sharing and validity, and replicability issues. Adjerid and Kelley (2018) alerted us to the fact that measurement quality needs to be improved for rigorous scientific work with big data. It is important to note that 'more' data does not necessarily improve the quality of measurement in research. Woo, Tay, Jebb, and colleagues (2020) discussed three ways in which the validity of big data measurements can be evaluated:

a   *Response processes* (i.e., the congruence between the construct and the nature of response engaged in by participants). This is an area where close collaboration between computer scientists (with skills to analyse sensor data) and sport scientists (with theories and understandings of human performance and expertise) will be useful for making sense of what information is valuable, where technology has to go to create valuable information, and what observed patterns actually mean.

b   *Internal (factorial) structure.* Studies with sensors have typically used single indicators, or the indicators simply provide an operational measure (Chaffin et al., 2017). In these cases, metrics about the internal structure are not relevant. However, combining multiple indicators can capture more complex constructs (Woo, Tay, Jebb et al., 2020). In these cases, exploratory or confirmatory factor models can be specified and tested for goodness of fit. It is also important to consider whether indicators are reflective of underlying constructs or they are formative (Edwards & Bagozzi, 2000). Given that sensor data provides multivariate time series data, longitudinal or dynamic factor models have to be developed and implemented to validate the use of indicators over time, at time scales that are both manageable (in terms of handling and analysing the data) and appropriate for capturing the construct under consideration (Davids et al., 2014).

c *Nomological net relations to other variables.* For a given construct of interest, it is important to examine both convergent and divergent associations across a range of potentially relevant constructs (Woo, Tay, Jebb et al., 2020).

Reliability estimates can be calculated on various parts of the data analysis process. If measurements are based on the notation of observers (e.g., registering the number of passes in a team ball game), reliability can be calculated using typical interobserver reliability statistics (e.g., kappa, intraclass correlation coefficient). For data-driven features (e.g., types of passes in a team ball game), sets of data can be randomly sampled, and the extent to which results replicate (e.g., the same words are classified in the same category) can be assessed. Alternatively, the continuous data can be split across several time points, and correlations across time sets indicate the cross-time consistency (Woo, Tay, Jebb et al., 2020). Chaffin et al. (2017) recently examined the reliability of sensor data on the use of wearable sensors for capturing behavioural variables. They discriminated between two sources of measurement error: problematic sensitivity differences between sensors (e.g., sensor A may be slightly more sensitive than sensor B), and differences within the same sensor across time. Their study suggests that researchers have to be careful in making inferences about differences between individuals because these differences may arise due to differences in sensors themselves.

Grasping Big Data with Visual Analytics

Big data analytics leaves out relevant contextual information in statistically modelling the world, which is complex, multidimensional, and intricate. Decision-makers contextualize analytical results within the broader context of society, and may even go against the analytical results of software to seek more favourable broader impacts when considering aspects that are reflected in the analysis (Karimzadeh, Zhao, Wang, Snyder, & Ebert, 2020). Given the abundant statistically significant relationships in big datasets, the meaningful relationships should be identified by the analyst. Visual analytics provides interactive access, organization, detail on demand, and contextual information to help decision-makers find relevant patterns. Visual analytics enhances computational algorithms by incorporating humans' extensive experience and domain knowledge that cannot be collected in the data (Karimzadeh et al., 2020). The contextual framework that makes humans identify what is relevant or meaningful for a given domain is based on cultural and social background practices.

Graphic displays of data, when properly designed, are efficient at communicating information and can provide more accessibility to valuable information that is not evident from big data. Data visualization is a set of methods for graphically, quickly, and accurately displaying data in a way that is easy to apprehend, and has two main functions: exploration and explanation (Sinar, 2015). The exploratory function of data visualization can help decision-makers identify underlying relationships that are hidden in raw data. The explanatory function can help them compose, analyse, and investigate research questions (Song, Liu, Tang, & Long, 2020). The analytical understanding of data is the basis of data visualization, but equally important is the perceived aesthetics of data visualizations. Advancements in both hardware and software have enabled computers to store and analyse massive amounts of data that often have high dimensionality. Some complex algorithms, such as machine learning models, are designed to reduce the massive amounts of complex data to manageable sizes and dimensions, and predict future states. However, the complexity and, at times, lack of transparency of the algorithms result in humans being unable to understand and trust the results (Burrell, 2016). Visual analytics combines the experience, contextual information, and expertise of the human user with the power of human-guided computational analysis, which, in turn, enhances the human decision-making process. Visual analytics incorporates the principles of design and cognitive science to identify appropriate visual analogies for data or analytical results, with a strong emphasis on creating perceptually effective representations for each analytical task (Karimzadeh et al., 2020).

Big data visualization techniques are not inherently different from small data visualization techniques. Capitalizing in what is traditionally used with small data, it is common to remodel familiar visualizations and integrate them within broader visual analytics systems with more interactivity and linked views (Robinson, 2011). For instance, the same visualizations for summarization (e.g., bar graphs, pie charts, line graphs) are used for big data but with more interactive features that can render additional elements and details on demand. Innovative data visualizations are more common with unstructured novel data sources. Visual analytics enables the integration of various computational models with interactive user interfaces for generating simulation results that facilitate testing various what-if scenarios for decision-making. Users can visualize and manipulate intermediate and final scenarios for key decision points (Karimzadeh et al., 2020).

Design of Visual Analytics Systems

Tay, Jebb, and Woo (2017) highlight that the following four issues need to be carefully considered in the design of visual analytics systems: (a) identification (isolating and highlighting relevant data and patterns, and the relevant scale of analysis), (b) integration (combining different data sources and different models to reveal new insights), (c) immediacy (streaming, real-time, and time-sensitive data, identify important dynamic changes over time using both incoming and historical data), and (d) interactivity (to select, switch, swap, and combine different data types on visual interfaces to inductively uncover and identify new patterns). The field of visual analytics expands on previous work to assist researchers, analysts, and decision-makers in their use of data for effective discovery, monitoring, analysis, and decision-making (Song et al., 2020). These aspects enhance the utility and usability of visual analytics. Utility refers to the ability of the system to support users in completing the required tasks, and usability describes the ease of using the system, according to the analyst perception, in completing the same required tasks (Ellis & Dix, 2006). To ensure utility and usability of a system, visual analytics researchers usually adopt the user-centred design paradigm, and work closely with stakeholders (e.g., directors, managers, coaches, trainers, analysts) at various stages of design and development. User-centred design usually entails identifying the context of use, specifying requirements, and creating design solutions. Creating solutions is typically an iterative process in which multiple design ideas are presented to users (via sketches or actual implementations of the system), feedback is sought, and intermediate assessments are conducted, leading to refining the design and presenting the system again for more feedback (Song et al., 2020). After a system implementation is completed, researchers conduct final evaluations through various protocols (Ellis & Dix, 2006) to report on the usability and utility of the system for the particular objective and users.

Research in computational methods, visualization, and cognitive science can help advance visual analytics by finding solutions that leverage both machine computational power and human intelligence. This is important not only to visual analytics but also to computational methods because automated methods are also marked by the choices (and potentially biases) that humans introduce when designing algorithms, sampling data, and interpreting the results (Karimzadeh et al., 2020).

Processing Big Data by Means of Artificial Intelligence

Part of the power of big data comes from the potential for using artificial intelligence, in particular machine learning and deep learning, approaches to identify coherent patterns in the data. Importantly, human observers are needed in these processes to monitor automatically created results to determine which patterns are meaningful and which are random (Woo, Tay, Jebb et al., 2020).

Machine Learning

Machine learning methods are a collection of statistical methods with the goal of creating reliable and replicable prediction models from datasets that may have a large number of variables. With a large number of variables, traditional approaches, such as multiple regression, may not yield reliable models of what to expect. To handle the large number of variables efficiently, machine learning algorithms can be used to search the predictor space and highlight variables with explanatory power (see Chapters 5 and 6). The methods do not guarantee that an ideal model is found, but instead they can find a model that performs well under a variety of conditions. Given the exploratory nature of these approaches, internal cross-validation methods are needed to prevent overfitting. Overfitting occurs when the model fits too closely to a specific dataset, such that the model accounts for the unique features of the data, which makes the model less generalizable when applied to a new dataset (Grimm, Stegmann, Jacobucci, & Serang, 2020). Moreover, the large number of participants and variables makes it possible to split the data randomly into smaller samples, allowing some subsets to be used to train models and other subsets to be used to test those models, making it possible to replicate findings within the same study. The accuracy of automatic models can also be compared with human annotations of a subset of data, providing an additional indication of accuracy (Woo, Tay, Jebb et al., 2020). Machine learning approaches can be generally categorized into supervised or unsupervised learning methods (Alpaydin, 2009).

Supervised Machine Learning

In supervised learning, a model is trained with labelled data for different prediction tasks such as classification (e.g., pictures classified into 'inside the score area' or 'outside the score area' category) or regression. The goal of supervised learning algorithms is to find the relationships or structures in the input data that allow a model to generate pre-defined output labels. These outputs are determined according to training data. Training data includes examples for which input and output are known, usually through the process of human manual annotation of input data (e.g., labelling a picture with 'inside the score area'). The way the training data is sampled and the method using it is annotated influence the generated automated models and may introduce the sampler's bias, especially if such a sample represents a snapshot in time, space, or event type. Most important, training data that does not reflect the input-output known relations may lead to contrived results that may go unnoticed (unless the assumptions and results are visually displayed to users with domain knowledge), and any sampling, by nature, introduces the biases of the analysts (Wallgrün, Karimzadeh, MacEachren, & Pezanowski, 2018). Furthermore, dynamic phenomena, such as human behaviours, do not lend themselves to a unique training of a machine learning model because such characteristics change due to context and entanglement of actions. Models generated for one particular event, time, or place may not work as well in other events. Machine learning, like traditional data analysis, may not model human and social contexts that cannot be easily collected in data and, therefore, lacks the ability to generate the background that a human analyst can bring to sequences of events, their relationships, and their context. Once such context changes, machine learning algorithms still perform according to the initial model training, whereas humans can base their understanding on the existing model results but also draw the necessary connections with the new context, and make appropriate inferences or decisions (Karimzadeh et al., 2020). For example, during the COVID-19 pandemic, people changed their online consumer behaviour in a way that affected the artificial intelligence models of the sellers' websites (e.g., Amazon). Humans' pandemic behaviour caused glitches for the algorithms related to inventory management, fraud detection, and marketing, among others. Many machine learning models trained on normal human behaviour could not predict nor classify behaviour (Heaven, 2020).

Unsupervised Machine Learning

This approach does not require labelled data or pretrained models. Instead, the training algorithm directly learns from the current data. For example, the K-means clustering algorithm finds the natural categories of data by maximizing 'within-cluster' similarity and minimizing 'inter-cluster' similarity (Karimzadeh et al., 2020). It can be used, for instance, to identify clusters of points scored in a volleyball match (i.e., the natural grouping of points that are similar to each other). Still, K-means requires the knowledge of the number of clusters (information that humans with domain knowledge easily have, even in the case of some unsupervised methods that can identify the optimum number of clusters). For example, the computer-generated clusters may be shifted significantly if outliers exist in the data. Again, decision-makers, if equipped with these tools, visuals, and information, are more reliable in identifying flawed outliers or natural extreme values depending on the context. Regardless of whether supervised or unsupervised methods are used, human involvement can ensure relevant results for changing context or dynamic phenomena. Visual analytics provides the infrastructure for human experts to adjust input and architecture (e.g., model configurations and structure), monitor a model performance (for precision or speed), compare results against reality and context, and improve the generated output labels to provide real-time examples for online learning (Karimzadeh et al., 2020).

Deep Learning

Deep learning is a specific type of artificial neural network with many layers (thus called 'deep') that has partly been revitalized due to recent advancements in hardware (LeCun, Bengio, & Hinton, 2015). Specifically, input values (e.g., pixel values in images) are multiplied by weights and added many times with constants to generate the desired (known) output values (e.g., digit labels for images containing 'inside the score area'). Deep learning relies heavily on large amounts of training data. The gold standard (currently most valid) examples are used in optimizing the weights and constants in the neural network and generating a model that can predict labels for the 'testing' data with acceptable accuracy levels. Testing data also usually is manually annotated by observers to ensure that the generated models can produce labels for examples that were not used during the training phase of optimization. Deep learning models require a high number of training examples for acceptable outputs (much higher compared with machine learning), given that many weights and constants in all the layers have to be optimized. However, training and testing data may only represent a snapshot of a time, space, phenomenon, or event. Building up a new representative training dataset is costly and laborious and, again, would only capture the variation of the world made on hard assumptions of sampling at the time. In certain scenarios, deep learning alone may suffer from the inability of decision-makers to adjust input parameters dynamically (to account for what-if scenarios of dynamic phenomena that need flexible inputs), detaching results from the context, and being specific to the training data instead of accommodating spatial or temporal variability in the phenomenon (Karimzadeh et al., 2020). Unlike traditional statistics, deep learning models are not geared for 'explaining' the relative importance or significance of input parameters, and therefore, deep learning models are not 'explanatory'. For instance, a simple linear regression model can explain the contribution of the 'number of completed passes' or 'shots on target' (as independent variables) to the 'teams winning a competitive match' (as the dependent variable). After the regression model is solved, the analyst can examine the generated coefficients and statistical significance values of independent variables and infer how much a unit increase, for instance, in the number of shots on target, would translate into a decrease (or increase) in expected match outcomes and if that value is in fact meaningful. Deep learning models, however, primarily focus on predicting the number of match wins without directly explaining the relative contribution of independent variables. This poses a problem for decision-makers and policymakers who do not just have to use the classification system, but have to understand the underlying phenomenon for planning and decision-making (Karimzadeh et al., 2020).

Machine Learning and Behaviour Recognition

Machine learning techniques can summarize a sequence of activities (Gandomi & Haider, 2015). Humans can usually recognize movement behaviours that are recorded in video images. However, it is more difficult to create computer software to perform such recognition processes. Behaviour recognition usually involves the following steps: (1) segmentation (classification of pixels), (2) motion detection (discrimination between pixels that are moving from those that are not), (3) object classification (classifies objects as humans or not), and

(4) motion tracking (follows objects from one frame to another) (Gowsikhaa, Abirami, & Baskaran, 2014). Motion detection, object classification, and motion tracking are all low-level processing techniques that are currently all machine based (i.e., involving machine learning algorithms). By contrast, behaviour recognition (pose, event, or activity recognition), behaviour analysis (spatial and temporal constraints, and semantic descriptions), and behaviour classification (number of persons interacting) are high-level processing techniques that can be either machine or human based because they are not yet fully automated (see Aghajanzadeh, Jebb, Li, Lu, & Thiruvathukal, 2020). Despite decades of research, many challenges remain in the automatic recognition and prediction of human behaviour by computer programs. Human behaviours have to be understood within a context. This context may or may not be easily determined from where the behaviour occurs. For example, people fighting on a street may be anomalous if it is related to social violence. However, fighting is expected in the event of a city martial arts demonstration. In this case, the location itself does not provide enough context to interpret the behaviour. The second challenge is that many applications require understanding of individual's behaviour in crowds when many other people are moving, which computer programs cannot do alone (Aghajanzadeh et al., 2020).

Although advanced analytic methods for big data serve as powerful tools to solve sport problems, they are not the solution for all cases. Researchers have to carefully examine the problem and data at hand to determine the most appropriate algorithm(s), instead of directly applying algorithms from previous research or practice. The choice of unsuitable methods makes it difficult to interpret results or, worse, leads to mistaken conclusions. Further, issues associated with overfitting could arise when a complex algorithm captures the training data too well, and the solution for the training data does not generalize to other datasets (Song et al., 2020). Moreover, big data analytics is developing rapidly, with new or refined algorithms and tools being continuously developed. It is both a challenge and an opportunity to re-evaluate statistical training to adapt to the world of big data.

Big Data and Sport Sciences: How to Converge?

Big data is intuitively appealing to sport scientists and practitioners because traditionally sports professionals and organizations have been major consumers of the large bands of data used to detect patterns and phenomena and yield more accurate estimates of performance and practice behaviours. Yet, these same big datasets may introduce new issues such as the way data are collected and cleaned, the type of hardware used, the expertise of the researcher, and the choice of analytic techniques (Adjerid & Kelley, 2018; Song et al., 2020). It is unsurprising that there are important methodological and empirical questions on the reliability, validity, and utility of big data for sport sciences. For example, there is limited evidence to date that machine learning algorithms can improve our ability to predict the outcomes of interest such as injury, winning, losing, or scoring (see Chapter 2). Going beyond the prediction accuracy, another notable problem with using machine learning algorithms in talent identification is the perpetuation of potential biases in the assessment and decision-making processes (cf. Güllich et al., 2019). These potential problems in assessment, prediction, and bias apply broadly to a vast array of sport sciences research and have to be better understood and clarified (Woo, Tay, & Proctor, 2020). Big data may also continue to underrepresent certain demographic groups, and analyses on subgroup differences may not be as robust. Also, there is the inevitable association of big data with lack of privacy and digital surveillance. Where data are being collected at scale without informed consent for a specific research question, there are questions such as when and how these types of data can be used, to what extent informed consent is necessary, and how the privacy of individuals can be protected in the analytic and research process. The emergence of such data requires sport scientists to work through ethical challenges of confidentiality and privacy related to big data (Woo, Tay, & Proctor, 2020). Song and colleagues (2020) believe more data security concerns will be addressed in institutional review boards. They rightly claim that it is our responsibility as researchers and practitioners to keep ourselves informed of the legal and ethical concerns, while advancing our knowledge and practice through the exciting promises of big data.

Another key concern for sport sciences is related to the loss of theoretical depth and specificity when big data advocates a preference for atheoretical procedures. Sport scientists are concerned with using data not only to maximize one's ability to predict meaningful outcomes but also to develop and further elaborate theories that provide meaningful explanations for observed relationships in performance, practice, and development (Araújo & Davids, 2016; Couceiro, Dias, Araújo, & Davids, 2016). However, new explanations from big data and artificial intelligence seem to be rare in practice. It may be due to the complex interactions between players, as it happens in team sports, and the lack of theory informing the use of methods. For example, the inconsistency of how events are identified, how the pitch zones are functionally defined, or how actions are seen in a context where attacking and defending co-exist impairs the reproducibility of studies within sport sciences (Passos, Araújo, & Volossovitch, 2017).

Abductive Method in Sport Sciences Research

Big data tends to be seen as an empirical paradigm that analyses large datasets for correlations between variables, rather than to be used to understand causes, preferring an inductive rather than hypothetico-deductive method, and eschewing theories that support scrutiny of potential causal mechanisms for performance and development. By privileging inference (instead of deduction), the inductive method has often been associated with narrow, short-term forms of thinking that contrive researchers to stay close to the observed data. The hypothetico-deductive method, preferred by the majority of sport scientists, pays closer attention to testing hypotheses and examining conceptual and theoretical relevance. The abductive method, with its emphasis on explanatory reasoning, is tailor-made for theorizing about performance aspects that tend not to be evident in observable phenomena (Haig, 2020). In fact, Haig (2020) proposes that the abductive method offers a useful framework for a broad array of big data research because it guides not only the initial process of phenomena detection (on which the inductive method focuses), but also the subsequent efforts towards theory construction where researchers generate, develop, and appraise theories. Importantly, Haig warns against the perspective, which assumes that big data analytic techniques allow the data to speak for themselves in a theory-free manner. Researchers should not confuse the identification of patterns in large datasets with interpreting, with reliability and validity, what these patterns may mean for understanding athlete performance and development.

For an abductive method, data-driven research leads beyond data patterns and empirical generalizations to explanatory hypotheses about the patterns of interest extracted from the data. Abductive inference is explanatory inference, and it involves reasoning about hypotheses, models, and theories in a manner that explains the relevant facts. Guided by evolving research problems that comprise packages of empirical, conceptual, and methodological constraints, sets of data are analysed in order to detect robust empirical regularities or phenomena. Once detected, these phenomena are explained by abductively inferring the existence of underlying causal mechanisms responsible for their production. Here, abductive inference involves reasoning from phenomena, understood as presumed effects, to their theoretical explanation in terms of underlying causal mechanisms (Haig, 2020). Theory informed (but not derived) methods (from an abductive inference paradigm) are not concerned with the testing of theories but with the formation of theories that arise out of data-analytic work (Haig, 2020).

More generally, inductive, abductive, and hypothetico-deductive theories of a scientific method can each be used to help meet their appropriate and different research goals in both big and small datasets about a given research problem. Inductive methods play an important role in the detection of empirical phenomena, different abductive methods combine to enable the construction of explanatory theories, and a hypothetico-deductive method can be used to test knowledge claims produced by the implementation of big data research strategies. A pluralist attitude to big data research, which allows different conceptions of causation to operate, is needed to contribute to the variety of causal claims made in science (Haig, 2020). Sport sciences tend to be mainly problem-oriented, where problems in performance, development, and preparation call for many solutions.

Big data allows research to capture various details of individuals' environments, often in a continuous manner, which can be used by sport scientists to analyse information structure in the environment, and how it constrains and guides performers (Davids, Handford, & Williams, 1994; Araújo, Davids, & Hristovski, 2006). However, the fact that the amount of data is 'big' does not necessarily mean that the data are better for research purposes or representative of the entire user population for the research question. The datasets collected in representative situations tend to reduce the control of variables, as typically happens in hypothetico-deductive research of human behaviour. Also, the *in situ* datasets are not necessarily random and are prone to issues like missing data due to the difficulties of the data collection process (Proctor & Xiong, 2020).

To date, computer scientists, engineers, and data scientists have been the main forces driving the development of how big data are coded, stored, and protected. Yet, the potential of big data needs to be recognized and exploited by other disciplines. To extract meaningful information from the increasingly large amounts of data, data visualization techniques have been developed. The work with big data seems to indicate that interdisciplinary work should be key for sport scientists to understand the information present in such sets. For this to occur, the goals of sport science should be highlighted for effective use, and appropriate conceptual language and analytical tools have to be formalized. Sport scientists themselves will need to develop and refine a good understanding of what value they may get out of big data if they are to contribute to theoretical understanding of sport phenomena. Sport scientists should play a major role in developing the language and tools of big data and how to communicate those effectively to coaches, practitioners, athletes, administrators, managers, and other stakeholders.

From Artificial Intelligence to Empowered Human Intelligence

Almost seven decades ago, computer pioneering Alan Turing suggested that digital computers, programmed with rules and facts about the world, might exhibit intelligent behaviour (Dreyfus, 1992). The field later called 'artificial intelligence' was about to be born. Many attempts, promises, failures, and successes emerged after that (Bostrom, 2017/2014). Bostrom (2017/2014), in his influential book on machine intelligence, defines 'superintelligence' as 'any intellect that greatly exceeds the cognitive performance of humans in virtually all domains of interest' (p. 26). He clarifies with the example of the chess program Deep Fritz. For him this program is not a superintelligence, because it is only smart within the narrow domain of chess. Therefore, for a machine to have general intelligence it needs to have the capacity to learn, to deal efficiently with uncertainty by means of calculating probabilities, to extract useful concepts from 'sensory input' and from its own internal states, and to leverage 'acquired concepts into flexible combinatorial representations for use in logical and intuitive reasoning' (p. 27). Interestingly, he emphasizes 'machines are currently far inferior to humans in general intelligence' (Bostrom, 2017/2014, p. 26).

In fact, a key part of his book is about speculating what are the paths to achieve superintelligence in the future.

Conceptual Problems with the Term 'Artificial Intelligence'

Dreyfus (1992, 2007) is less optimistic that 'it is just a matter of time to develop artificial intelligence'. For Dreyfus, the core assumption of artificial intelligence that human beings produce intelligence using facts and rules seems to have compromised the entire artificial intelligence (AI) research programme. The main problem is that of representing significance and relevance, based on the assumption that the mind assigns value to a world conceived as a set of meaningless facts. The key difficulty is that attributing functions to cold facts could not capture the meaningful organization of the everyday world. Beyond the difficulty of storing myriads of facts about the world, the main problem is knowing which facts are relevant in a given situation (see Dreyfus, 1992): when something in the world changes, how does the program determine which of its represented facts can be assumed to have stayed the same, and which might have to be updated? One answer offered by AI researchers to this problem was to use a frame, or a structure of essential features and default assignments. But a system of frames does not belong to the analysed situation, so in order to identify the possibly relevant facts in the current situation one would need a frame for recognizing that situation, and so forth. Therefore, there is an infinite regress of frames for recognizing relevant frames for recognizing relevant facts.

The early 'Good Old-Fashioned Artificial Intelligence' systems developed by Herbert Simon and colleagues, based on the physical symbol system approach, got trapped in this infinite regress (Bostrom, 2017/2014; Dreyfus, 1992). Other recent approaches such as neural network modelling tried to avoid it, by means of giving sufficient examples of inputs associated with one particular output, to associate further new inputs with the 'same' output. But there is still the problem of what qualifies as 'same' needs to be defined by the programmer. S(he) has determined, by means of the architecture of the net, that certain possible generalizations will never be found. In daily life, a large part of human intelligence consists in generalizing in ways that are appropriate to a context. If the programmer restricts the net to a predefined type of correct responses, the net will be exhibiting the intelligence built into it by the programmer for that context but will not have the intelligence that would enable it to adapt to other contexts.

Human Intelligence

The key point is that using pre-established rules, facts, and sequential operations is not how humans typically express their expertise, because skilled performance implies background context, skills, and openness to a dynamic situation (Rietveld, Denys, & Van Westen, 2018; Woo, Tay, Jebb et al., 2020). Intelligence seems to emerge from human intentionality and goals picked up by a moving person in an ongoing culture. Everyday background practices, as Dreyfus (2007) put it, allow humans to experience what is currently relevant as they deal with things and people. It is *knowing of* the world, and not only *knowing about* the world, that characterizes intelligent behaviour and performance in sport (Araújo, Cordovil, Ribeiro, Davids, & Fernandes, 2009). This *knowledge of* the world is based on the history of interactions with contexts, events, and people, along with the unique characteristics, body, needs, and skills of each person (Araújo, Dicks, & Davids, 2019). It is hard to disclose how to convey such knowledge to a computer. Skills for dealing with events and people are different from facts about them, which can be stored digitally in a kind of coded list from which the program selects which facts that match the situation and those that do not. These models imply that the programmer select fixed (predefined) features about the world which serve as an input for the program, and then design the criteria for a successful output. However, in performance and everyday life, humans interact directly with the world, a world that is not fixed and where context matters. The world is its own best model, indicating that it is not how humans represent it internally that matters, but how the world is presented to the person and how the person with his/her unique characteristics perceives and acts in a dynamic world that characterizes intelligence (Araújo, Hristovski, Seifert, Carvalho, & Davids, 2019; Dreyfus, 2007; Merleau-Ponty, 1945). Embodied, sentient beings like humans take as input energy from the physical universe but do not attribute meaning to this energy; humans do not see the reflected light, but they see objects and people. Instead they respond in a way as to open themselves to a world organized in terms of their needs and bodily capacities – without their minds needing to impose meaning to meaningless 'sensory input', nor their brains converting stimulus input into pre-programmed responses. When performing, individuals are not experiencing objects, surfaces, or people as such, they are simply acting upon the possibilities or affordances they offer in the performance environment (Gibson, 1979). Such affordances disclose the world on the basis on which we sometimes do step back and perceive objects, surfaces, or people as such. But the way humans solve problems is by being drawn in by an 'inviting affordance' (Withagen, de Poel, Araújo, & Pepping, 2012). Affordances are experienced as a solicitation that calls for a flexible response to the current situation, improving it or making it worse. Our experience feeds back and changes our sense of significance for the next situation and what is relevant in that next situation. This relevance is not determined beforehand, because if it was, humans could not respond to new relevant opportunities (Dreyfus, 1992).

Intelligent Sport Performance

An intelligent performer in sport contexts is a highly adaptive individual. The dynamical interactions of an athlete with a performance environment help him/her detect information from different perceptual modalities and guide decision-making and actions (Button, Seifert, Chow, Araújo, & Davids, 2020). The ecological dynamics approach stresses the primacy of establishing functional individual-environment relations in understanding intelligent behaviour. Studying the couplings formed between a performer and a performance environment helps us to understand complex aspects of human behaviour in the actual world such as moving around, selecting paths, or deciding with whom to cooperate and compete. In this view, any system that is capable of successfully engaging in such dynamic events exhibits intelligence. From this perspective, cognition is embodied and embedded so that perceiving an event with its temporal and spatial characteristics specifies body forces and torques required in goal-directed action. If intelligence is understood as something separated from the body and the environment, it denies that major influences operating on most cognitive systems are from the social and physical environment (e.g., Araújo et al., 2010), as well as from their own action-perception skills (Araújo, Hristovski et al., 2019).

Intelligent behaviours are understood and necessarily constrained by the evolving environment-individual system. The current state of this system is the result of a history of interactions that constrains the immediate action. In this way, current performance is continuously shaped by previous interactions. An individual's behavioural history channels action to a landscape of possibilities for behaviour (affordances). The precise place in the affordance landscape that a performer is guided towards emerges according to the particular history of each individual in many contexts. The affordance landscape reflects the multiple possibilities for action that stand out as relevant for each individual in a particular situation because of specific training, skills, and experience in related tasks (Rietveld et al., 2018). This means that the behavioural landscape is constrained by goals, intentions, motivations, and needs towards which actions may be directed as well as the environment that draws the individuals into it and solicits actions. Intelligent behaviour is constrained by both its history and its prospective implications. Action is an ecologically flexible process (self-organized, emergent). Intelligent actions that emerge in a performance environment are holistic entities that are different from the components that make up the system (e.g., the field, the ball, performer's legs) and cannot be predicted solely from the characteristics of those components. Consequently, many sorts of solutions to a sport problem can emerge given the many ways its elements can interact under the same constraints. But instead of being a random process, or, in the other extreme, a process that is internally programmed in advance, performers are perceptively attuned to affordances from the context that guide self-organizing action towards achieving (or not) a task goal (Davids & Araújo, 2010). The dynamic process implied in the perception of affordances provides the basis by which a performer can (self) regulate his/her behaviour prospectively. Intelligence, therefore, should be understood not in terms of discrete mental operations, combining rules with facts, but in terms of the self-regulating relationship that emerges between individuals and their environment in striving to achieve an intended task goal (Araújo et al., 2006; Withagen, Araújo, & de Poel, 2017).

Intelligent Sport Performance Is Embodied

For understanding human intelligence, there is a need to emphasize the importance of understanding the role of the body. As Merleau-Ponty (1945) argued, to move one's body is to aim at things through it, it is to allow oneself to respond to the solicitation of things, which is made upon it independently of any internal representation. In human skilled activity, performers are drawn to move so as to achieve a better familiarity and proneness to respond to the situation. Acting is a continuous responding, guided by perceptual attunement, to the situation. Action is also a means to move to better perceive (anticipate) what to do next (Gibson, 1979; Stepp & Turvey, 2010). When a performer's situation deviates from some body-environment relationship, his/her activity re-takes him/her closer to an equilibrium informed by the deviation from such state. Given our experience, whenever there is a change in the current situation, the performer responds to it based on how his/her experience become built in his body, how the body as a whole developed over time, and when (s)he senses a significant change, (s)he treats everything else as unchanged except what his/her attunement to the situation suggests might also have changed and so needs to be adjusted. With experience, affordances become perceptually salient (perceptual attunement) and simply elicit what needs to be done (perception-action coupling). Our familiarity enables us to respond to what is relevant and ignore what is irrelevant without planning based on purpose-free representations of context-free facts (Dreyfus, 1992). Once we are in a situation without representing it, the problem of priority of context and facts, that AI is facing, does not arise.

A brain alone might still not be able to respond to new sorts of situations because our ability to be in a situation might depend not just on the flexibility of our nervous system but rather on our ability to engage in perceptual-motor activity. As Dreyfus (1992) aptly synthesized 'it might become apparent that what distinguishes persons from machines, no matter how cleverly constructed, is not a detached, universal, immaterial soul but an involved, situated, material body' (p. 236). In short, humans must be understood in more diverse terms than simply their nervous system. Humans are active beings, where intentionality, understood as directness towards objects, structures experience. A machine can possibly make a specific set of hypothesis and then find out if they have been confirmed and refuted by data. The body can constantly modify its intentionality in a flexible way, because it needs not to check for specific characteristics, but simply for whether it is coping with the situation (Dreyfus, 1992). Dreyfus argues that coping need not be defined by any specific set of features but rather by an ongoing mastery to maintain a stable relationship with the situation. What counts as a stable relationship varies with the goal of the performer and the resources of the situation. Thus, it cannot be expressed in context-free and purpose-fixed terms.

If one thinks of the importance of the perceptual-motor skills in the development of our ability to perceive and act upon the situation, or of the role of intentionality and needs in structuring social situations, or of the whole cultural background involved in performers' *knowing of*, formalizing their understanding as a complex system of facts and rules is highly questionable. In other words, human intelligence is based on the role of the body in organizing and unifying our experience of objects, events, and people, the role of the situation in providing a background against which behaviour can be orderly without being rule-like, and the role of human intentionality in organizing the situation so that the objects are recognized as relevant and accessible (Dreyfus, 1992).

Ecological Dynamics Approach Informs the Use of Artificial Intelligence in Sport

Ecological dynamics construes that goal-directed behaviours in sports emanate from the hard-assembled (physical) and soft-assembled (informational) links between performers and their performance environments (Kugler & Turvey, 1987). This idea implies that ecophysical variables (Araújo, Davids, & Renshaw, 2020) provide the most appropriate starting point to capture intelligent behaviour (see Chapter 3). These are variables that express the fit between the environment and the performer's adaptations. As mentioned before, environmental properties may directly inform what an individual can and cannot do (Withagen et al., 2012). For example, Fink, Foo, and Warren (2009) demonstrated (by manipulating the trajectories of fly balls in a virtual environment) that how a performer gets to the right place at the right time to catch the ball is solved by relying on a strategy of cancelling optical acceleration (of the image of the ball on the catcher's eyes). The strategy of moving in order to cancel the ball's optical acceleration exemplifies how each player's change in movement can be defined intrinsically by the player's relationship with the environment (Harrison, Turvey, & Frank, 2016). The vertical optical acceleration of an approaching object can provide time-to-collision information without the need to mentally compute either distance or speed of the object to intercept it (Michaels & Zaal, 2002). An important challenge for researchers and practitioners using artificial intelligence is to capture ecophysical variables in their work to enable understanding of how intelligent behaviour might be predicated on perception-action couplings during continuous, emergent, performer-environment interactions in sports.

To sum up, for artificial intelligence to empower human intelligence, an ecological dynamics approach offers at least three suggestions. First, the sources for big data can emphasize ecophysical variables. More than the traditional emphasis in personal characteristics (e.g., height), accumulated performances (e.g., number of assists last season), or even environmental variables (e.g., size of the birth city, number of spectators), the emphasis could be placed on how the performer interacts with the circumstances of performance as captured by ecophysical variables (e.g., Carrilho et al., 2020). Second, visual analytics is highly encouraged as a tool for interpreting the data, where its display can be developed in an interdisciplinary way, with the contribution of sport scientists and practitioners, computer and data scientists, and engineers (Couceiro et al., 2016). Visual analytics and carefully developed infographics may be well placed to consider the context, in a way that an automated, context-free, output may never offer. Finally, the computation behind the analysis of big data is clearly a process that arises from the domain of expertise of computer scientists. Sport scientists typically do not have the background to programme such algorithms. However, the joint work about how the data can be analysed may fruitfully develop variables and their treatment that may better consider relevant aspects of the sport under consideration (e.g., Araújo & Davids, 2016; Couceiro et al., 2016). Moreover, given the expertise of sport scientists to understand how movement, body, and context contributes to understand intelligent performance behaviours, they can work together with computer scientists in developing less mentalist, and more embodied and embedded, architectures for capturing the impact of artificial intelligence. This is the purpose of this book.

2

HOW IS ARTIFICIAL INTELLIGENCE BEING USED IN THE SPORT SCIENCES TO ANALYSE AND SUPPORT PERFORMANCE OF ATHLETES AND TEAMS?

Introduction

Artificial intelligence (AI) is having a huge impact in society in general, and specifically in the scientific community (Ertel, 2017; Kubat, 2015; Muazu Musa et al., 2019; Pappalardo et al., 2019). In sport, over the past decades, coaches and practitioners have been using statistics and data analytics in an extensive way – in an attempt to measure any aspect of athlete behaviour, on- and off-field – that can be quantified. Aligned with this trend, AI is becoming an important tool to help coaches to make better decisions and to manage different problems (Bianchi, Facchinetti, & Zuccolotto, 2017). Nevertheless, the effective application, interpretation, and use of data in some behavioural contexts are still under question (Claudino et al., 2019), requiring further development by the AI community with regard to athlete development and performance preparation in sport (Lam, 2018).

It is well known that advanced performance analytics in contemporary high-performance sports can help support staff, sport scientists, and practitioners confront different problems (Bianchi et al., 2017). Artificial intelligence has been broadly conceptualized as the study of how to support computers to perform operations and tasks, at which, currently, people are better (Rich, 1983), with the definitive goal of understanding intelligence and building intelligent systems to improve organization and function of systems in daily life (Ertel, 2017).

The human dream that machines would one day be able to learn how to perform basic functions and tasks, currently undertaken by people, has existed for many generations. Machine learning is a field of AI which has been characterized as the study of computer algorithms that allow computer programs to automatically improve through experience (Mitchell, 1997). In other words, machine learning is an area of computer science that aims to teach computers how to learn from patterns in large sets of data and act beyond the initial program designed by a computer scientist (Samuel, 1959, Chapter 1).

There is a growing interest in applying machine learning algorithms to different examples of human performance behaviours by explicitly deriving models based on probabilistic reasoning (Lam, 2018). Campaniço, Valente, Serôdio, and Escalera (2018) proposed that the study of the effectiveness and efficiency of an athlete's performance can be supported by technology implementation, providing coaches and practitioners with invaluable tools for the treatment and analysis of massive volumes of statistical information (*big data*, see Chapter 1) with relative ease.

From an applied point of view, machine learning is a powerful tool for classification and prediction (Chapters 5 and 6). In a simplistic way, these models take a selection of certifiable evidence (features) and predict what that evidence represents (Whiteside, Cant, Connolly, & Reid, 2017). Well-developed analytical techniques can benefit many interested professionals, including sports team managers and administrators needing evidence for making recruitment and planning decisions, the coaches and support staff, and the athletes themselves (Lam, 2018). What does existing research tell us about the implementation of AI and machine learning algorithms in the preparation of athletes for sport performance? What are the trending research topics in these areas? How are these engineering methods being applied in understanding how to enhance athlete performance? These are the questions this chapter addresses.

AI in Sport Science: Research overview

To provide relevant insights on the important athlete and team performance issues that AI and machine learning methods are currently being used to investigate, this chapter provides a systematic review of the available literature. This literature review was conducted according to PRISMA (Preferred Reporting Items for Systematic Reviews and Meta-Analyses) guidelines (Moher, Liberati, Tetzlaff, & Altman, 2009). The electronic databases Web of Science, Pubmed, and SPORTdiscus were searched for relevant publications prior to the 10th of March 2020 by using the keywords: ('machine learning' OR 'predictive modelling' OR 'learning algorithms' OR 'data mining' OR 'deep learning' OR 'artificial intelligence' OR 'extreme learning machines') AND ('team sport*' OR 'sport*' OR 'performance'). Publications included in the first selection round met the following criteria: (1) contained relevant data concerning AI, (2) were performed on individual/team sports, and (3) were written in the English language. Studies were excluded if they: (1) did not contain any relevant data about AI and sports, and (2) were reviews or conference abstracts.

Two reviewers independently screened citations and abstracts to identify articles potentially meeting the inclusion criteria. For those articles, full text versions were retrieved and independently screened by the reviewers, to determine whether they met specified inclusion criteria. In line with good practice in methodologies for systematic reviews, any disagreements regarding study eligibility were resolved by consensus involving a third reviewer.

The initial search identified 2,143 titles in the aforementioned databases. These data were then exported to reference manager software (EndNote™ X9, Clarivate Analytics, Philadelphia, PA, USA). Any duplicates (796 references) were eliminated either automatically or manually. The remaining 1,347 articles were then screened for relevance based on their title and abstract, resulting in 1,084 studies being eliminated from the database. The full text of the remaining 263 articles was examined in more detail and 192 were rejected because they did not meet the inclusion criteria. At the end of the screening procedure, 71 articles were selected for in-depth reading and analysis (Figure 2.1). The main factor for study exclusion from this specific review ($n = 112$) was their lack of relevance to the research topic. Other studies were excluded because they were conference abstracts ($n = 57$) or written in other languages than English ($n = 23$).

To adopt a global view of what research is telling us about the use of AI in understanding sport performance, we grouped the studies according to the most common research topics in individual and team sports. The results showed that the body of scientific research at this time has focused mainly on: (1) predicting performance, (2) injury prevention, and (3) pattern recognition (Figure 2.2).

Current AI research in team sports has been centred mainly on understanding these topics in specific modalities like football (American, Australian, and

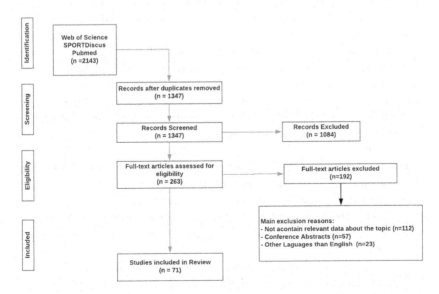

FIGURE 2.1 Preferred reporting items for systematic reviews via flow diagram.

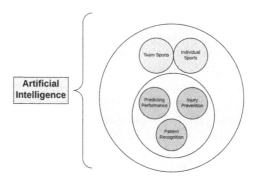

FIGURE 2.2 Scopes of AI in sports performance.

Association/soccer), basketball, volleyball, and rugby. Undoubtedly soccer is the sport that has received the most attention from researchers, perhaps reflecting the funding available for implementation of these technologies. Although rarer, studies on baseball, ice hockey, futsal, archers, biathlon, cycling, fencing, golf, skateboarding, skiing, swimming, tennis, and table tennis were also found (Tables 2.1 and 2.2). In the next section, we evaluate research findings concerning the main issues investigated, as reflected in Figure 2.2.

Predicting Performance

Our analysis of past performances and the prediction of future performances, published in peer-reviewed research journals and outlets, have revealed a number of interesting tendencies that can help athletes and teams in their training processes. With the rapid advance in science and technology, specifically using sophisticated data mining and AI algorithms, forecasting the outcome of a specific competitive event is becoming more feasible (Cheng, Zhang, Kyebambe, & Kimbugwe, 2016). A central goal of sports statistics and analytics is to understand patterns and actions, which may be closely related to gaining a successful competitive outcome. As sports organizations have entered the world of big data, there is an increasing opportunity for large-scale AI methods to model complex sports performance dynamics (Schulte et al., 2017). This type of predictive analysis has been targeted by the scientific community to seek for the best methods that make it possible to predict the outcome of a specific competitive event or game or to identify for selection the creativity of developing players (Memmert & Perl, 2009a, 2009b). It is notable that both these major aims are likely to yield the greatest financial benefits for technological applications.

For example, Delen, Cogdell, and Kasap (2012) concluded that classification-type models predict the outcomes of American football games better than regression-based classification models, and of the three classification techniques used

TABLE 2.1 Summary of studies on AI in team ball sports

	Sport	Sample	Aim	Machine learning models	Conclusions
Delen et al. (2012)	American football	Data from eight sporting seasons of NCAA	To predict the outcome of a college football game	Decision trees, neural networks, support vector machines	The results showed that the classification–type models predict the game outcomes better than regression-based classification models, and of the three classification techniques, decision trees produced the best results, with better than an 85% prediction accuracy on the ten-fold holdout sample
Bock (2017)	American football	32 teams spanning seven full seasons	To test if turnovers were predictable	Gradient boosting machines (GBMs)	Under certain conditions, both fumbles and interceptions can be anticipated at low false discovery rates (less than 15%)
Cai et al. (2018)	American football	58 reconstructed head impacts include 25 concussions and 33 non-injury cases	To develop a deep learning approach for concussion classification	Support vector machine (SVM), random forest (RF), and univariate logistic regression	This study demonstrates the superior performances of deep learning in concussion prediction and suggests its promise for future applications in biomechanical investigations of traumatic brain injury

(Continued)

	Sport	Sample	Aim	Machine learning models	Conclusions
Bergeron et al. (2019)	American football and other contact sports	Data from three years of concussions (n = 2004) suffered by high school student-athletes in football and other contact sports	To implement a supervised machine learning–based approach to model if estimated symptoms evolve over time in high school athletes who incurred a concussion during sport activity	Logistic regression, naïve Bayes (NB), SVM, 5-nearest neighbours (5NN), C4.5 decision tree (C4.5D and C4.5N), random forest (RF100 and RF500), multilayer perceptron, and radial basis function network	Supervised machine learning demonstrated efficacy, while warranting further exploration, in developing symptom-based prediction models for practical estimation of sport-related concussion recovery in enhancing clinical decision support
Ruddy et al. (2018)	Australian football	Data from 362 players	To investigate the predictive ability of hamstring strain injury risk factors using machine learning techniques	Naïve Bayes, logistic regression, random forest, support vector machine, neural network	Risk factor data cannot be used to identify athletes at an increased risk of hamstring strain injury with any consistency
Robertson et al. (2019)	Australian football	9,005 kicks from the 2015 Australian Football League	To develop working models for the determination of high frequency, representative events in Australian Rules football kicking	Rule induction models, random forest (RF)	When considering the relationships and interaction between constraints and skilled performance, rule induction provides a method capable of reducing the complexity of large datasets without compromising its inherent structure

Reference	Sport	Data	Aim	Method	Findings
Ross, Dowling, Troje, Fischer, and Graham (2018)	Baseball	Data from 542 athletes performing seven dynamic screening movements	To determine if principal component analysis could detect meaningful differences in athletes' movement patterns when performing a non-sport-specific movement screen	Principal component analysis and linear discriminant analysis	The authors proved that an objective data-driven method can detect meaningful movement pattern differences during a movement screening battery based on a binary classifier (i.e., skill level in this case)
Chen, Chou, Tsai, Lee, and Lin (2012)	Baseball		To propose an HMM-based ball hitting event exploration system for broadcast baseball video	Hidden Markov models	Convincing results and encouraging performance are obtained when compared with previous existing baseball video systems
Bhandari et al. (1997)	Basketball	Row data from NBA	To describe Advanced Scout software from the perspective of data mining and knowledge discovery	Attribute focusing	The process of pattern interpretation is facilitated by allowing the user to relate patterns to video tape
Schmidt (2012)	Basketball	Data from 21 participants that performed (each one) 20 free-throw trials	To analyse the movement patterns of free-throw shooters in basketball at different skill levels	Neural networks (Dycon)	A high stability of the network methods was documented

(Continued)

	Sport	Sample	Aim	Machine learning models	Conclusions
Kempe et al. (2015)	Basketball	Positional data of ten players during a game	To investigate the ability of merge self-organizing map to analyse spatio–temporal data and compare its performance to the common dynamical controlled network approach to analyse team sport position data	Neural networks	The authors concluded that introduced SOMs can be easily trained with tracking data of one or more teams and automatically classify the conducted actions in real time
Lopez and Matthews (2015)	Basketball	Predictors for NCAA basketball tournaments (e.g., final score at home and away matches, distance travel in away matches)	To analyse the accuracy of traditional methods vs cutting-edge predictive algorithms	Logistic regression and log– loss function	The use of informative data with traditional statistical tools can still result in predictions whose accuracy rivals that of more complex models
Cheng et al. (2016)	Basketball	Data from 14 basic technical features from all games of 2007–2008 season to 2014–2015 season	To predict the outcome of National Basketball Association (NBA) matches	Maximum entropy model, k-means clustering, naïve Bayes, logistic regression, BP neural networks, random forest	Overall, the NBA Maximum Entropy (NBAME) model is able to match or perform better than other machine learning algorithms

(Continued)

Bianchi et al. (2017)	Basketball	Data from 82 games of 2015–2016 NBA regular season	To describe new roles of players during the game	Neural networks (self-organizing maps, fuzzy clustering)	When considering the modern basketball players' statistics, classical positions are not able to fully represent their way of playing, and a new set of five roles emerges as a meaningful classification of players' characteristics
Leicht et al. (2017)	Basketball	Women's basketball matches during the 2004–2016 Olympic Games ($n = 156$)	To examine the relationship between team performance indicators and match outcome during the women's basketball tournament at the Olympic Games	Binary logistic regression, conditional interference classification tree	Incorporation of non-linear analyses may provide teams with superior/practical approaches for elite sporting success
Lam (2018)	Basketball		To model two-team sports for the sake of one-match-ahead forecasting	Bayesian regressions	85.28% of the matches in NBA 2014/2015 regular season were correctly predicted by TLGProb (two-layer gaussian process regression model for winning probability calculation), surpassing the existing predictive models for NBA

	Sport	Sample	Aim	Machine learning models	Conclusions
Schulte et al. (2017)	Ice hockey	Data from SportLogiq, which contains over 1.3 million events in the National Hockey League	To develop a context-aware approach to valuing player actions, locations, and team performance in ice hockey	Markov game	Model validation shows that the total team action and state value both provide a strong indicator predictor of team success, as measured by the team's average goal ratio
Jäger and Schöllhorn (2007)	Volleyball	Data from the first round of the 2002 women's World Volleyball championship in Munster, Germany	To develop a classification of offensive and defensive behaviours and to identify team-specific tactical patterns in international women's volleyball	Hierarchical cluster analysis	This approach to team tactical analysis yields classifications of selected offensive and defensive strategies as well as an identification of tactical patterns of different national teams in standardized situations
Jaeger and Schoellhorn (2012)	Volleyball	120 standard situations of six national teams in women's volleyball are analysed during a world championship tournament	To identify different team tactical patterns in volleyball and to analyse differences in variability	Artificial neural networks	The results showed that defence systems in team sports are highly individual at a competitive level and variable even in standard situations. Artificial neural networks can be used to recognize teams by the shapes of the players' configurations

Gomez, Herrera Lopez, Link, and Eskofier (2014)	Volleyball	Present methods for the determination of players' positions and contact time points by tracking the players and the ball in beach volleyball video	To present and compare two methods for the determination of players' positions and contact time points by tracking the players and the ball in beach volleyball videos. Two player tracking methods were compared	Classical particle filter and a rigid grid integral histogram tracker	In this study, tracking results of over 90% from the literature were not to be confirmed
Hsu, Chen, Chou, and Lee (2016)	Volleyball	97 volleyball rallies	To develop a novel 2D histogram-based player localization method capable of locating players with occlusions	Histogram based-approach vs connected component analysis and histogram of oriented gradient	The experiments on broadcast volleyball videos demonstrate efficient and effective results against a traditional object segmentation method (connected component analysis) and a supervised learning approach utilizing histogram of oriented gradient features

(Continued)

	Sport	Sample	Aim	Machine learning models	Conclusions
Passos et al. (2006)	Rugby	Responses of 32 different dyads performed by eight male rugby players (11–12 years of age)	(1) To identify phase transitions in a team ball sport with task constraints different from those of basketball; (2) to present a 3D analysis of interpersonal dynamics of attacker–defender dyads; (3) to identify parameters to measure dynamical systems properties in these dyads	Artificial neural networks	The results confirmed that artificial neural networks are reliable tools for reconstructing a 3D performance space and may be instrumental in identifying pattern formation in team sports generally
Passos et al. (2008)	Rugby	Responses of 48 different dyads performed by eight male rugby players (11–12 years of age)	(1) To determine how interpersonal coordination patterns in attacker–defender dyads, exemplifying outcomes such as tries or tackles, emerge in performance; (2) to study pattern-forming dynamics in different team sports and to identify relevant order and control parameters that accurately describe dyadic system behaviour under distinct performance task constraints	Artificial neural networks	The results suggested that relative velocity increased its influence on the organization of attacker–defender dyads in rugby union over time as spatial proximity to the try line increased

Kelly, Coughlan, Green, and Caulfield (2012)	Rugby	Data from 1,179, 619, and 383 impacts peaks were detected for player A, B, and C, respectively	To investigate tackle modelling techniques which can be utilized to automatically detect player tackles and collisions	Support vector machine and hidden conditional random field	The results of the validation showed that the system is able to consistently identify collisions with very few false positives and false negatives
Chambers, Gabbett, and Cole (2019)	Rugby	Data from 30 elite rugby players: 46 matches and 51 training sessions	To investigate whether data derived from wearable microsensors can be used to develop an algorithm that automatically detects scrum events in rugby union training and match play	Random–forest classifier-based algorithm	The scrum algorithm was able to accurately detect scrum events for front-row, second-row, and back-row positions
Jonsson et al. (2006)	Football	Data from six games from the Spanish La liga	To present a new approach to the study of actions between players in team sports	T-pattern	The results showed that it is possible to identify new kinds of profiles for individuals/teams on the basis of observational criteria and a further analysis of temporal behavioural patterns detected within the performances

(Continued)

	Sport	Sample	Aim	Machine learning models	Conclusions
Joseph et al. (2006)	Football	Data from 1995/1996 and 10996/1997 Tottenham Hotspur Football Club sporting seasons	To predict the outcome (win, lose, or draw) of matches played by Tottenham Hotspur Football Club	Bayesian networks; MC4, a decision tree learner; naïve Bayesian learner; data-driven Bayesian (a BN whose structure and node probability tables are learnt entirely from data); k-nearest neighbour learner	The ability of Bayesian networks to provide accurate predictions without requiring much learning data is an obvious bonus in any domain where data are scarce
Min et al. (2008)	Football	Data from two teams that participate in the world cup	To develop a framework for sports prediction using Bayesian inference and rule-based reasoning, together with an in-game time-series approach	Bayesian networks	The authors have implemented a football results predictor called FRES (Football Result Expert System) based on this framework, and shown that it gives reasonable and stable predictions
Martinez-del-Rincon et al. (2009)	Football	Data from 20 players form two soccer teams	To develop a complete application capable of tracking multiple objects in an environment monitored by multiple cameras	Bayesian estimation	The developed system is satisfactory and shows a substantial improvement over systems based on manual labelling. This system allows processing a complete match in a few hours using a conventional laptop

Motoi et al. (2012)	Football	Data from 40-dimensional sequences extracted from real professional soccer games	To develop a method for soccer game event detection with an HMM in a hierarchical Bayesian framework	Bayesian HMM	The developed algorithm appears to be functional
Grunz et al. (2012)	Football	Data from the soccer world championship final 2006	To find tactical patterns in those positional data	Artificial neural network	The results showed that short and long game initiations can be detected with relative high accuracy leading to the conclusion that the hierarchical architecture is capable of recognizing different tactical patterns and variations in these patterns
Leo, Mazzeo, Nitti, and Spagnolo (2013)	Football		To present a new approach to recognizing soccer ball instances in images acquired from static cameras	Multi-step algorithm	The effectiveness of the proposed methodologies has been demonstrated through a huge number of experiments using real balls under challenging conditions, as well as a favourable comparison with some of the leading approaches from the literature

(Continued)

	Sport	Sample	Aim	Machine learning models	Conclusions
Montoliu et al. (2015)	Football		To use a new technology to perform team pattern recognition and analysis in football	Neural network multilayer perceptron, distance–based classifier k-nearest neighbour, the learning–based classifier support vector machine, the ensemble learning–based classifier random forest	The proposed methodology is able to explain the most common movements of a team and to perform the team activity recognition task with high accuracy when classifying three football actions: ball possession, quick attack, and set piece. Random forest is the classifier obtaining the best classification results
Arndt and Brefeld (2016)	Football	Data from five seasons (2009/10–2013/14) of the German Bundesliga	To propose a multitask, regression–based approach for predicting future performances of soccer players	Multitask regression (ridge regression and support vector regression)	The proposed multitask generalizations of ridge regression and support vector regression allowed efficiently learning player-specific models
Brooks et al. (2016)	Football	Data from 2012–2013 La Liga season	To analyse pass event data to uncover sometimes-nonobvious insights into the game of soccer	K–nearest neighbour, support vector machine	The authors showed that appropriate analyses of pass-event data in soccer can provide interesting and sometimes nonobvious insights

| Sarmento et al. (2016) | Futsal | Data from 126 goals scored of 30 games and 17 individual players | To quantify the type of offensive sequences that result in goals in elite futsal | T-pattern analysis | T-pattern analysis of offensive sequences revealed regular patterns of play that are common in goal scoring opportunities in futsal and are typical movement patterns in the sport |
| Chawla et al. (2017) | Football | Data from four matches played in the English Premiership during the 2007/08 season (2,932 passes) | To produce an automated system to evaluate the quality of passes made between players during the game | Multinomial logistic regression, support vector machine (SVM) classifier, and a RUSBoost classifier | Experimental results demonstrated that the system is able to produce a classifier with 85.8% accuracy on classifying passes as Good, OK, or Bad, and that the predictor variables computed using complex methods from computational geometry are of moderate importance to the learned classifiers |

(Continued)

	Sport	Sample	Aim	Machine learning models	Conclusions
Constantinou and Fenton (2017)	Football	Data from several European teams (league points, injuries, European competitions, managerial changes, promoted teams)	To develop a model that generates accurate predictions of the evolving performance of football teams based on limited data	Time-series forecasting	The model enables the prediction, before a season starts, of the total league points a team is expected to accumulate throughout the season. Additionally, the model results provide a comprehensive attribution study of the factors most influencing change in team performance, and partly address the cause of the widely accepted favourite-longshot bias observed in bookies odds
Link and Hoernig (2017)	Football		To describe models for detecting individual and team ball possession in soccer based on position data		

Martins et al. (2017)	Football	Match results from the different championships: English Premier League (EPL), season 2014/2015; La Liga Primera Division (LLPD), season 2014/2015; and Brazilian League Championships, seasons 2010 (BLC 2010) and 2012 (BLC 2012)	To develop a new approach to predict matches' results of championships	Polynomial classifier in association with: naïve Bayes, decision tree, multilayer perception, radial basis function, and support vector machine	The association between polynomial algorithm and machine learning techniques allowed a significant increase of the accuracy values. The presented polynomial algorithm provided an accuracy superior to 96%, selecting the relevant features from the training and testing set
Razali et al. (2017)	Football	Data from the English Premier League for the seasons of 2010–2011, 2011–2012, and 2012–2013	To present a Bayesian networks to predict the results of football matches in terms of home win, away win, and draw	Bayesian networks	Bayesian networks achieved predictive accuracy of 75% in average across three seasons. The results could be used as the benchmark output for future research in predicting football matches results

(Continued)

	Sport	Sample	Aim	Machine learning models	Conclusions
Schlipsing, Salmen, Tschentscher, and Igel (2017)	Football		To present a real-time system acquiring and analysing video sequences from soccer matches	Linear discriminant analysis (LDA), nearest neighbour (NN), and one-vs-all multi-class support vector machines (SVMs)	The authors concluded that: (1) deliberate use of machine learning and pattern recognition techniques allowed us to achieve high classification accuracy in varying environments; (2) a proper human machine interface decreases the number of required operators who are incorporated into the system's learning process
Barron et al. (2018)	Football	Data from 966 outfield players, each completing the full 90 minutes from 1,104 matches played in the English Football League Championship during the 2008/09 and 2009/10 seasons	To identify key performance indicators in professional soccer that influence outfield players' league status	Neural network	The findings of this study have shown that it is possible to identify performance indicators using an artificial neural network that influences a players' league status and accurately predicts their career trajectory

Cho et al. (2018)	Football	Data from UEFA Champions league press kits data	To present the conceptual framework of a soccer win–lose prediction system focused on passing distribution data	Social network analysis, gradient boosting vs support vector machine, neural network, decision tree, case-based reasoning, logistic regression	The results and analyses demonstrate that the network indicators generated through social network analysis can represent soccer team performance and that an accurate win–lose prediction system can be developed using gradient boosting technique
Jaspers et al. (2018)	Football	Data from 38 professional soccer players over two seasons	To evaluate the ability of machine learning techniques to predict the RPE of soccer training sessions from a set of external load indicators	Artificial neural network, least absolute shrinkage and selection operator (LASSO)	Both the artificial neural network and LASSO models outperformed the baseline. In addition, the LASSO model made more accurate predictions for the RPE than did the artificial neural network model
Pappalardo and Cintia (2018)	Football	Data from more than 6,000 games and 10 million events in six European leagues	To quantify the relation between performance and success	Ordinary least squares regression	The simulation produces a team ranking which is close to the actual ranking, suggesting that a complex systems' view on soccer has the potential of revealing hidden patterns regarding the relation between performance and success

(Continued)

	Sport	Sample	Aim	Machine learning models	Conclusions
Rossi et al. (2018)	Football	Data from 26 Italian professional male players during season 2013/2014	To develop a multi-dimensional approach to injury forecasting in professional soccer that is based on GPS measurements and machine learning	Forecast model	The study showed that the forecaster can be profitably used early in the season, and that it allows the club to save a considerable part of the seasonal injury–related costs
Takahashi, Yokozawa, Mitsumine, and Mishina (2018)	Football	4,500 images of balls. Video sequences of 900 consecutive frames	To develop a robust ball-position measurement system that can be used for actual football games	Support vector machine	The proposed system can robustly measure the position of a football in real time and is effective for producing live football broadcasts
Geurkink et al. (2019)	Football	Data resulting from 61 training sessions, and 913 individual training observations were obtained	To predict the session Rate of Perceived Exertion (sRPE) in soccer and determine the main predictive indicators of the sRPE	Gradient boosting machines	The results showed that the sRPE can be predicted quite accurately, using only a relatively limited number of training observations
Pappalardo et al. (2019)	Football	Data from four seasons of 18 prominent soccer competitions	To design and implement PlayeRank, a data-driven framework that offers a principled multi-dimensional and role-aware evaluation of the performance of soccer players	Linear support vector classifier	The results showed that PlayeRank is an innovative data-driven framework that goes beyond the state-of-the-art results in the evaluation and ranking of soccer players

TABLE 2.2 Summary of studies on AI in individual sports

Muazu Musa et al. (2019)	Archers	50 youth archers with the mean age and standard deviation of (17.0 ± 0.56) years drawn from various archery programmes completed a one end archery shooting score test	To classify and predict high and low potential archers from a set of physical fitness variables trained on a variation of k-NN Algorithms and logistic regression	k-nearest neighbour, multiple linear regression agglomerative cluster analysis	The k–nearest neighbour outperformed all the tested models and it demonstrated reasonably good classification on the evaluated indicators with an accuracy of 82.5 ± 4.75% for the prediction of the high–potential archers and the low potential archers
Maier, Meister, Trösch, and Wehrlin (2018)	Biathlon	Data from 118,300 shots from four seasons	To explore factors influencing biathlon shooting performance and to predict future hits and misses	Logistic regression model, tree-based model with boosting, and an artificial neural network	To predict future shots, a simple machine learning model using only an athlete's preceding mode-specific hit rate showed some predictive power. Nevertheless, a high degree of randomness involved in every shot persisted, which complex models could not substantially reduce

(Continued)

Ofoghi, Zeleznikow, MacMahon, and Dwyer (2013)	Cycling	Data from senior riders of different world championships	To describe the implementation of machine learning techniques that assist cycling experts in the crucial decision-making processes for athlete selection and strategic planning in the track cycling omnium	Cluster analysis (k-means clustering algorithm) naïve Bayes	The study indicates that sprint events have slightly more influence in determining the medallists, than endurance-based events. Using a probabilistic analysis, the authors created a model of performance prediction that provides an unprecedented level of supporting information that assists coaches with strategic and tactical decisions during the omnium
Campaniço et al. (2018)	Fencing	Data from two exercises performed 1,000 and 700 times respectively in two daily sessions, by a single fencer	To explore the technical optimization of an athlete through the use of intelligent system performance metrics that produce information obtained from inertial sensors associated to the coach's technical qualifications in real time	Artificial neural network	The performance analysis of the resulting models returned a prediction accuracy of 76.6% and 72.7% for each exercise, but other metrics indicate the existence of high bias in the data

Couceiro, Dias et al. (2013)	Golf	Data from six expert golf players	To analyse the golf putting performed by expert players, using an algorithm that automatically detects stationary and dynamic objects	Linear discriminant analysis, quadratic discriminant analysis, naïve Bayes with normal distribution, naïve Bayes with kernel smoothing density estimate, least squares support vector machines	The authors concluded that the five pattern detection methods used (with different levels of performance) can be applied to the study of coordination and motor control on the putting performance, allowing for the analysis of the intra- and interpersonal variability of motor behaviour in performance contexts
Corrêa et al. (2017)	Skateboarding	543 artificial acceleration signals	To explore the state of the art for inertial measurement unit use in skateboarding trick detection, and to develop new classification methods	Artificial neural networks	Machine learning can be a useful technique for classifying skateboarding flat ground tricks, assuming that the classifiers are properly constructed and trained, and the acceleration signals are pre-processed correctly
Rindal et al. (2018)	Skiing	24 datasets from ten different participants	To optimize the accuracy of the automatic classification of classical cross-country skiing sub-techniques by using two inertial measurement units attached to the skier's arm and chest together with a machine learning algorithm	Neural network	Overall, the authors achieved a classification accuracy of 93.9% on the test data. Furthermore, they illustrate how an accurate classification of sub-techniques can be combined with data from standard sports equipment including position, altitude, speed and heart rate measuring systems

(Continued)

Nemec et al. (2014)	Skiing	Data from five highly skilled skiers (two females and three males)	To propose two machine learning methods that overcome this shortcoming and estimate centre of mass and skis trajectories based on a more faithful approximation of the skier's body with nine degrees of freedom	Neural networks, statistical generalization	The results outperform the results of commonly used inverted-pendulum methods and demonstrate the applicability of machine learning techniques in biomechanical measurements of alpine skiing
Mezyk and Unold (2011)	Swimming	Data collected in two months (February–March 2008), among swimmers from swimming sections in Wrocław	To use a machine learning approach combining fuzzy modelling with an immune algorithm to model sport training	Fuzzy-based data mining	The proposed machine learning tool acquires the rules from the dataset on the level of almost 70% accuracy
Xie et al. (2017)	Swimming	Data concerning 4,022,631 swim records	To investigate performance features for all strokes as a function of age and gender	KNN, linear-SVM, RBF-SVM, DT, RF, AdaBoost, NB, LDA, Quadratic discriminant analysis, quadratic polynomial regression, ANN, and support vector regression	The simulation experiments demonstrate that the new method combining multiple inference methods to derive Wisdom of Crowd Classier (WoCC) is a consistent method with better overall prediction accuracy. The study reveals several new age-dependent trends in swimming and provides an accurate method for classifying and predicting swimming times

Lim, Oh, Kim, Lee, and Park (2018)	Table tennis	Data from two table tennis players on five table tennis skills: forehand stroke, backhand drive, backhand short, forehand cut, forehand drive	To present a deep learning-based coaching assistant method, which can provide useful information in supporting table tennis practice	Combination of long short-term memory with a deep state space model and probabilistic inference	The experimental results showed that the developed method can yield promising results for characterizing high-dimensional time-series patterns and for providing useful information when working with wearable IMU (Inertial measurement unit) sensors for table tennis coaching
Lai et al. (2018)	Table tennis	Data from 723,057 table tennis matches played by 21,458 players in Italy in five seasons	To estimate the contribution of the network of matches in predicting an athlete's success	Combining network analysis and machine learning	Results showed that machine learning approaches are able to predict players' success and that the topological features play an effective role in increasing their predictive power
Lara Cueva and Estevez Salazar (2018)	Tae Kwon Do	Data from 76 athletes	To develop a system based on the information of the classification for the athletes in Tae Kwon Do	Decision tree and support vector machines	The proposed novel support system can be useful to determine the suitable athletes for the next competitions in this sport, while giving a robust and operative overview of features for athletes' selection management purposes

(Continued)

	Sport	Data	Aim	Method	Findings
Kovalchik and Reid (2018)	Tennis	Data from one of the sport's four Grand Slams (2015–2017 Australian Open)	To establish a complete shot taxonomy for professional men's and women's tennis using spatiotemporal data	Multi-stage model-based clustering approach	Results showed that shot type was strongly associated with winning points and shots in the highest speed and lowest net clearance categories tended to be the most effective
Bacic and Hume (2018)	Tennis	43 swings were recorded in one session by a certified tennis coach (the first author) under guidance of another certified international tennis coach	To develop a proof-of-concept prototype combining kinesiology and artificial intelligence that could help improving tennis swing technique	Evolving clustering method	The developed prototype demonstrated autonomous assessment on future data based on learning from prior examples, aligned with skill level, coaching scenarios, and coaching rules
Whiteside et al. (2017)	Tennis	Data from 18 athletes wore an inertial measurement unit (IMU) on their wrist during 66 video-recorded training sessions	To develop an automated stroke classification system to help quantify hitting load in tennis	Support vector machine, discriminant analysis, random forest, k-nearest neighbour, classification tree, neural network	The combination of miniature inertial sensors and machine learning can offer a practical and automated method for quantifying shot counts and for discriminating shot types in elite tennis players

Kovalchik et al. (2017)	Tennis	Data from 86 ATP and 82 WTA matches from the 2016 Australian Open	To investigate decision-making with the use of the challenge system	Recursive partitioning decision tree	Ball and player location were the most important factors for successful challenge. Players could use challenges more effectively and tennis stakeholders could improve the integrity of the system by taking steps to reduce delayed challenges and impact bias among chair umpires
Panjan et al. (2010)	Tennis	1,002 male and female tennis players who had undergone regular testing by the Slovenian National Tennis Association	To examine the predictability of the competitive performance of tennis players by using the most promising morphological measures and motor tests selected by automatic computer methods and by experienced tennis coaches	Naïve Bayes classification method, decision tree, the C4.5 algorithm, the k-nearest neighbour, support vector machine, and logistic regression	The results revealed that automatic methods for identifying the most promising variables proved to be more successful than those of the coaches, which was most clearly noticeable with regard to the female tennis players and when linear regression was used
Ida, Fukuhara, Sawada, and Ishii (2011)	Tennis	Data from eight experienced and eight novice players rated their anticipation of the speed, direction, and spin of the ball on a visual analogue scale	To determine the quantitative relationships between the server's motion and the receiver's anticipation using a computer graphic animation of tennis serves	Multiple regression analyses	The results showed that the experienced players demonstrated a higher coefficient of determination than the novice players in their anticipatory judgement of the ball direction

(Continued)

| Memmert and Perl (2009a) | Multidimensional | 42 children | To present a new neural network approach for analysis and simulation of creative behaviour | Artificial neural networks | The results showed that the network is able to separate main process types and reproduce recorded creative learning processes by means of simulation |
| Memmert and Perl (2009b) | Multidimensional | 20 soccer players, 17 field hockey players, and 18 individuals in a control group | To develop a framework for analysing types of individual development of creative performance based on neural networks | Artificial neural networks | The authors concluded that by using neural networks it is now possible to distinguish between five types of learning behaviour in the development of performance |

(decision trees, neural networks, and support vector machines), decision trees produced the best results. However, in basketball, Cheng et al. (2016) concluded that the NBA Maximum Entropy (NBAME) model is able to at least match or outperform other machine learning algorithms. Additionally, Lopez and Matthews (2015) advocated that traditional statistical tools can still result in predictions with accuracy levels that rival those of more complex models. Also Leicht, Gomez, and Woods (2017) examined the relationship between team performance indicators and match outcome during women's basketball matches ($n = 156$) through linear (binary logistic regression) and non-linear (conditional interference classification tree) statistical techniques. They identified that shooting proficiency and defensive actions of individuals were key team performance indicators in the analysed teams. The findings highlighted the usefulness of incorporating non-linear analyses in order to provide sports organizations with superior approaches for performance preparation in seeking elite sport success. More recently, Lam (2018) proposed a pioneering modelling approach (sparse spectrum Gaussian process regression) based on stacked Bayesian regressions. In their work, the author modelled sports by associating the players' abilities with teams' strengths using stacked regressions and concluded that 85% of the matches in NBA 2014/2015 regular season were correctly predicted by two-layer gaussian process regression model for the winning probability calculation, surpassing the existing predictive models for NBA.

Soccer is the sport with the greatest number of published AI analyses. In some studies, researchers tried to predict competitive match outcomes using Bayesian networks (Joseph, Fenton, & Neil, 2006; Min, Kim, Choe, Eom, & McKay, 2008; Razali, Mustapha, Yatim, & Ab Aziz, 2017), and these models showed reasonable and stable predictions. Additionally, the results showed that the expert Bayesian networks are generally superior to other techniques for this domain in predictive accuracy. Time forecasting (Constantinou & Fenton, 2017), naïve Bayes, decision tree, radial basis function, support vector machine, and social network analysis (Cho, Yoon, & Lee, 2018; Martins et al., 2017) have also been used. The understanding that coaches and practitioners can gain from the machine learning process allows the development of models, which reflects what we have learned from research about the relationships between the attributes (28 players, performance venue, and opponent quality – 30 attributes in total) and the relative importance of each attribute. Specifically in soccer, it enables us to see which of the selected attributes are the crucial factors in predicting the outcome of a game, providing some clues as to the relationships between some of those factors (Joseph et al., 2006). According to Joseph et al. (2006), when approaching a new problem there are two techniques which are commonly used: (1) as we have an idea how the situation under investigation works, we construct a model, and using this model we select the attributes believed to contribute to the effect under investigation; (2) we assume little knowledge of the underlying mechanisms involved, so we look at all the probably relevant attributes and try to determine those which have the most significant effect. The prediction of match outcomes is a very difficult problem because there are too many unpredictable variables, such as the relative weaknesses/strengths of either team, the existence of injured players, players' attitudes, and team managers' operations that influence who may win (Cheng et al., 2016).

In addition to trying to predict the outcomes of a game, there is a set of other articles that seek to analyse more specific aspects related with the performance of teams and athletes. For example, Bock (2017) tested if the turnovers in American football are predictable. Bearing in mind that a positive differential turnover margin in a given game is a significant predictor of winning that game, the author applied the gradient boosting machines technique and concluded that both fumbles and interceptions can be anticipated at low false discovery rates (less than 15%). In sport sciences, these analyses are important, since the ability to anticipate catastrophic in-game events may lead to better management and control, ultimately improving the performance of athletes/teams (Bock, 2017).

According to Araújo, Davids, and Serpa (2005), representative learning design provides a framework to the extent to which practice as preparation for competition simulates key elements of a performance setting. In this sense, Robertson, Spencer, Back, and Farrow (2019) presented a different approach using rule induction, to develop working models for the determination of high frequency, representative events in Australian Rules football kicking. They concluded that rule induction provides a method capable of reducing the complexity of large datasets without compromising its inherent structure. Additionally, the results showed that it could be used to quantitatively define events within a representative learning design framework.

Moreover, some investigators have applied the neural network methodologies in different ways, such as: (i) to describe new roles of players during a basketball game (Bianchi et al., 2017), (ii) to produce an automated system to evaluate the quality of passes made between players during a soccer game using multinomial logistic regression, support vector machine classifier and a RUSBoost classifier (Chawla, Estephan, Gudmundsson, & Horton, 2017), and (iii) to predict the soccer career trajectory of individual players (Barron, Ball, Robins, & Sunderland, 2018). A different approach was presented by Jaspers et al. (2018) and Geurkink et al. (2019) who predicted the Rate of Perceived Exertion (RPE) in soccer players using artificial neural networks, LASSO, and gradient boosting machines. The applied machine learning techniques revealed to be valuable to predict RPE values for future sessions and may help a coaching staff to plan, monitor, and evaluate training sessions.

Studies developed in the context of individual sports are focused mainly in the application of machine learning techniques to predict performance. For example, in table tennis (Lai, Meo, Schifanella, & Sulis, 2018), taekwondo (Lara Cueva & Estevez Salazar, 2018), and archery (Muazu Musa et al., 2019), machine learning techniques were applied to classify and predict the potential of the athletes. In the three sports, the tested models proved to be efficient in predicting: (1) high-potential archers, (2) table tennis players' success and that the topological features play an effective role in increasing their predictive power, and (3) the most suitable athletes for the next competitions in taekwondo. Bearing in mind that talent identification and development is an area where sports organizations currently invest significant funding, the integration of these analytical techniques can become an important tool in the future. Additionally, in skateboarding (Corrêa, Lima, Russomano, & Santos, 2017), skiing (Nemec, Petric, Babic, & Supej, 2014; Rindal, Seeberg, Tjonnas, Haugnes, & Sandbakk, 2018), tennis (Bacic & Hume, 2018; Kovalchik & Reid, 2018; Kovalchik, Sackmann, & Reid, 2017; Panjan, Šarabon, & Filipčič, 2010; Whiteside et al., 2017), and swimming (Mezyk & Unold, 2011; Sadeghizadeh, Saranjam, & Kamali, 2017; Xie, Xu, Nie, & Nie, 2017), there is a growing interest in the application of machine learning techniques for the study of particular aspects of athletes' performance (e.g., shot types in tennis players, factors influencing biathlon shooting performance, exploration of the technical optimization in fencing) that can help shape the training and preparation processes. One example of this adaptation of the training process emerged from the results of the study by Mezyk and Unold (2011), which collected data from swimmers' training sessions for two months and developed an algorithm that proved to be efficient to identify the accurate training stimulus in an appropriate timescale for each athlete in preparation for competition.

Injury Prevention

Although sport injuries have long been recognized as a global health problem and a priority area by some local and national government agencies, there is still scarce information on the patterns of incidence of sports injuries at a broad level in most countries.

Injury incidence is an important aspect in sport practice. In team sports, athletes' performance availability has a strong correlation with team success (i.e., ranking, position, games won, goals scored), and is also a financial burden to clubs (López-Valenciano et al., 2020). Taking soccer as an example, the average cost of a footballer in a professional top team being injured for one month is calculated to be around €500,000 (Ekstrand, 2013). In this sense, developing accurate and reliable injury predictors is a central aspect in the domain of sport sciences. Information from such systems could be closely aligned with preventative training measures to reduce likelihood of injuries during the busiest periods of a competitive season in team sports.

Rossi et al. (2018) developed a multi-dimensional approach to injury forecasting in professional soccer, based on GPS measurements and machine learning. The study showed that the forecasting system can be profitably used early in the season, and that it allows the club to save a considerable part of the seasonal injury-related costs. This approach opens a novel perspective on injury prevention, providing a methodology for evaluating and interpreting the complex relations between injury risk and training performance at a professional level in soccer.

Concussion prevalence in sport, and more specifically in American football, is well recognized (Bergeron et al., 2019). During the past years, there has been significant attention to sports-related concussions as a major cause of mild traumatic brain injury and athletes and parents have raised concerns about the causes and implications of concussions in professional and amateur sports leagues (Haider et al., 2018). In soccer, for example, there have been questions raised over long-term effects of heading a ball travelling at great speeds and there have been attempts to reduce heading frequency in children's games.

Cai et al. (2018) developed a deep learning approach for concussion classification using implicit features of the entire voxel-wise white matter fibre strains. Based on reconstructed NFL injury cases, leave-one-out cross-validation was employed to compare injury prediction performances against two baseline machine learning classifiers and four scalar metrics via univariate logistic regression. They concluded that feature-based machine learning classifiers including deep learning, support vector machine, and random forest consistently outperformed all scalar injury metrics across all performance categories. Additionally, Bergeron et al. (2019) implemented a supervised machine learning-based approach in modelling estimated symptom resolve time in high school athletes who incurred a concussion during sport activity. They suggested that supervised machine learning demonstrated efficacy in developing symptom-based prediction models for practical estimation of sport-related concussion recovery in enhancing clinical decision support.

Pattern Recognition

Pattern recognition is one of the areas where AI has had most impact over the past years. A set of studies has focused on pattern recognition (e.g., identification of tactical patterns, patterns of movement by individuals and sub-groups, interpersonal coordination patterns) or tracking systems (using, for example, 2D histogram-based player localization method, Bayesian HMM, support vector machine).

Sport performance behaviours imply successful tactics and strategies by players and teams, which can be analysed with the aim of identifying regular movement and interaction patterns during particular sequences (James, 2012). Classically, the underlying assumption for any prediction model is that performance is repeatable, to some degree. In this sense, there are attempts to detect patterns of play or movement in sport (Van Winckel et al., 2014). Several techniques have been used to identify movement patterns. A promising technique that has been recently employed in investigating common movement patterns in sports is T-pattern detection and analysis (TPA) that was initially based on behaviour organization theory and uses probability theory and an evolution algorithm. T-patterns can also be understood as probabilistic natural (pseudo) fractals recurring with statistically significant translation symmetry. The TPA algorithm now includes parallel processing. Using TPA, Sarmento et al. (2016) and Jonsson et al. (2006) verified the existence of regular patterns of play in futsal and soccer (respectively) that are common in leading to the emergence of goal scoring opportunities.

Using artificial neural networks, several investigators have tried to identify specific patterns of play in basketball (Bhandari et al., 1997; Kempe, Grunz, & Memmert, 2015; Schmidt, 2012), volleyball (Jaeger & Schoellhorn, 2012), soccer (Grunz, Memmert, & Perl, 2012; Montoliu, Martín-Félez, Torres-Sospedra, & Martínez-Usó, 2015), and rugby union (Passos et al., 2008; Passos, Araújo, Davids, Gouveia, & Serpa, 2006). Passos and colleagues (2006) analysed interpersonal coordination patterns in rugby and highlighted some practical advantages of artificial neural networks for analysing sport performance: (1) once the network for a specific performance field has been created, the only major concern is to locate the cameras at exactly the same place and height, to facilitate different types of movement analysis; (2) there is no need to know any of the intrinsic/extrinsic camera parameters, such as focal distance and camera position related to the origin; (3) when a sufficient number of reference points are used, results produced are accurate even in the presence of optical and/or digital distortion; and (4) taking into account that a set of points from a reference structure is needed for the training and validation procedures, the knowledge of certain kinds of measures that represent the depth, width, and height of the performance field (e.g., length of field lines, distance between lines) can provide a set of points large enough to feed the net for those procedures.

In addition, the application of hierarchical cluster analysis has allowed the identification of tactical patterns of different volleyball national teams in standardized situations (Jäger & Schöllhorn, 2007). Moreover, using supervised machine learning techniques (e.g., K-nearest neighbour, support vector machine), Brooks, Kerr, and Guttag (2016) built a model for predicting whether a sequence of passes by a team will end in a shot at goal in soccer, providing a map to understand the relative importance for generating shot opportunities of passing from one location to another.

A Highlighted Source of Big Data for Artificial Intelligence: The Growing Impact of Automated Tracking Systems

As seen in Chapters 1 and 3, machine learning has become increasingly popular in computer vision-based applications due to the state-of-the-art results reachable in the image classification, object detection, and natural language processing domains of performance (Elhoseny, 2020). Video watching applications are becoming increasingly important for analysing individual performance, and video object tracking is an essential task because it generates interrelated temporal data about the moving objects in a film clip (Luo et al., 2018). Over the last few years, systems capable of tracking the movement of players and the ball in different sports (e.g., football, rugby, handball) have multiplied, which provides a detailed characterization and analysis of the behaviour of athletes and teams.

The usefulness of this type of technology was well demonstrated by Chambers et al. (2019), who developed and validated a scrum algorithm to automatically detect scrum events in rugby. Such innovation allows a significant efficiency in the process of players' performance analysis, since previously, this type of analysis was only possible through the use of notational analysis techniques which proved to be very time consuming. Using automated tracking system technology and analysis allows coaches and sport scientists to determine the physical load associated with these contact events, which should improve player-training process and reduce the risk of injury.

In volleyball, Hsu et al. (2016) developed an automatic system capable of extracting play-by-play periods and locating players using a novel 2D histogram-based approach, which proved to be effective not only for obtaining tactical information but also for collecting descriptive performance statistics during competition. Additionally, Gomez et al. (2014) compared two player tracking methods (a classical particle filter and a rigid grid integral histogram tracker) in beach volley. They concluded that contrary to the previous literature where tracking results of over 90% were verified, in this study tracking accuracy of the ball was 54.2% for the trajectory growth method and 42.1% for the Hough line detection method. The difficulties in accurately detecting the ball trajectories had also been previously reported by Chen et al. (2012) in baseball, and by Leo et al. (2013) in soccer. More recently, Takahashi et al. (2018) reported to have a successful experience in improving a system to automatically detect the movement of the ball in soccer, integrating tracking results from multi-view cameras in real time.

Over the last decades there has been an exponential increase in soccer video analysis research (Leo et al., 2013). Using Bayesian methods, some investigators (Martinez-del-Rincon et al., 2009; Motoi et al., 2012) tried to develop some game tracking systems that have revealed some functionality in detecting in-game events. These models seem to be important not only for coaches and practitioners but also for an increasing number of fans at home or in the stadium who may be interested in consuming more 'live' detailed, performance information.

Conclusion

Research on AI in sports has been exponentially growing in the past ten years. Existing research has supported the identification of the most frequently addressed topics in this area of research both in individual and team sports:

(1) predicting performance, (2) injury prevention, and (3) recognition of patterns of play, and other specific sport actions.

Predicting performance is a central goal of sports analytics and statistical analyses with consequences for theory and practice. In the last few years, since sports organizations have entered the world of big data, there is an exponential growth in the AI applications to predict sports competition dynamics, with repercussions on how to prepare athletes and teams for performance. Several areas of progress have emerged over the last decade in order to understand, methodologically, which algorithms are more effective in predicting sport performance and injuries, or in developing automated performance tracking systems. Nevertheless, there is a need to develop this area – not only through the use of theoretically informed performance indicators that are representative of the dynamics of sports, but also through the contribution of coaches, athletes, and practitioners with their experiential knowledge to validate the relevance and the search for meaningful variables.

Video-based approaches and related data computation are an important technology for sport, allowing a drastic reduction in the number of hours of work that would normally be required to collect information manually. Besides all the potential benefits resulting from the application of AI to sport, the quality of the data is of paramount importance. In this sense, departments of methodology and theoretical informed practices need to be implemented to get full benefit of such algorithms.

Despite the recent increase in the application of AI in sports, there is still a large margin for development. In this sense, in the short term it will be possible to improve the information that is transmitted to the sport scientists, support staff, and coaches in real time, through the use of portable devices and software that allow practitioners to measure the activity of athletes and teams. Additionally, this information can be used more frequently for decision-making by coaches. Finally, the widespread use of these technologies may also facilitate better interaction with supporters, thus favouring the industry underlying sport.

3

FROM RELIABLE SOURCES OF BIG DATA TO CAPTURING SPORT PERFORMANCE BY ECOPHYSICAL VARIABLES

Representative Assessment Design and Technology

Technological advances provide the opportunity to further study and augment the understanding of the athletic performance as (i) they provide data that were not available in the past, and (ii) they allow computation of metrics that was not done in the past (see Chapter 1). For instance, machine and deep learning techniques allow overcoming the computation of 'low level' indicators to add 'high level' indicators (e.g., intra- and inter-team organization), which can be done along the matches and/or the training sessions. In order to quickly provide feedbacks to practitioners about the behaviours and performance of the athletes, technological advances developed new devices and new applications/ algorithms (e.g., embedded sensors like smartwatches, smartphones, global positioning system – GPS, often complemented with accelerometers, constituting inertial measurement unit – IMU) and new tracking systems, notably based on progress in computer vision (e.g., multi-camera motion capture, TV broadcast tracking, deep learning approaches to 3D markerless motion capture, RGB depth camera). One issue with technological advances is that sensors always provide some data to scientists and practitioners, even when those data are poorly collected, poorly reflecting the core of practice or reflecting a decontextualized or non-representative designed protocol for collecting data, confirming the weakness of data-driven approaches (Couceiro et al., 2016). Moreover, a second issue is to have too much data, which request scientists to data reduction or dimensionality reduction by using techniques from AI (e.g., machine or deep learning). These issues raise the problem of how data reduction and data modelling do not reduce information meaning for practitioners. Moreover, when fuzzing data, reducing dimensionality, and modelling data, the outcome is sometimes complex to understand and to interpret for the coach, in the sense that the transfer from data analytics to sport intervention is far from direct. These risks could be overcome by appropriately designing procedures for data acquisition, defining the assessment task, the data collection method, and relevant technology. We argue that appropriately designed methodologies should root in the ecological dynamics framework. One theoretical pillar of this framework refers to *perception-action coupling* (Araújo & Davids 2015; Araújo, Davids, & Passos, 2007) and emphasizes the importance of a *representative (experimental) task design* (Brunswik, 1956).

Brunswik (1956) proposed the term *representative design* to advocate the study of psychological processes at the level of organism-environment relations. It means that contextual variables should be sampled from the organism's environment so as to represent the environment where the organism behaves, and to which behaviour in the experiment is intended to be generalized. This definition of representative design emphasizes the need to ensure that learning, training, or experimental task constraints represent the task constraints of the performance or game/race environment that forms the specific focus of study. Representative design implies a strong emphasis on the specificity of the relations between the athlete and the environment, which could be neglected in data-driven approaches to behavioural sciences. The ability of performers to detect and use information from the environment to support their actions is predicated on an accurate and efficient relationship between perceptual and motor processes, referred to as *perception-action coupling* (Pinder, Davids, Renshaw, & Araújo, 2011a). For example, Dicks, Button, and Davids (2010) compared movement and gaze behaviours of soccer goalkeepers in a typical video simulation with *in situ* research designs. The authors showed significant differences between task constraints that required verbal or simulated movements compared with those realized *in situ*, performing interceptive actions when facing penalty kicks. Such findings suggest that high representativeness of learning/training design would capture the *perception-action coupling* as it happens in competition and promote skill transfer between the learning task and the competition. Moreover, this study also points out the required caution when using video support for learning, training, and performance analysis, which if not properly used may decouple perception from action. In another example, Pinder, Davids, Renshaw, and Araújo (2011b) emphasized the risk of using devices like ball projection machines, as they might remove remove key information sources from the performance environment (e.g., the movement of the bowler) and significantly affect the timing and control of interceptive actions in cricket batting. These authors observed significant differences between the practice task constraints, with earlier initiation of the backswing, front foot movement, downswing, and front foot placement when facing the bowler in contrast with facing the bowling machine. Therefore, more specific skill transfer may be expected when batting against a bowler bowling a ball (supported by the functional coupling between perception and action), while general skill transfer might occur when a bowling machine projects the ball. When using new technology for intervention and data collection, scientists and practitioners must be aware that this equipment might have an impact on the specificity of the skill transfer. Of course, when a bowling machine is used to project the ball, the reproducibility of the task is high and movement analysis can focus essentially on the batter. Conversely, when the bowler bowls the ball, movement analysis could also be directed to the bowler's actions, as the batter picks up information from the bowler. For this to happen, the motion capture systems need to comprise both the bowler and the batter, which could lead to very heavy data collection (e.g., huge volume to capture and calibrate, many body markers to assess accurately upper body and arm). Moreover, when scientists decide to perform in-depth microscopic analysis, it sometimes demands heavy, intrusive (for the athletes), and time-consuming equipment for setting of the motion capture systems (e.g., multi-optokinetic camera system), which might disturb the data collection or even the athlete motion. Therefore, to guarantee representative experimental design, scientists should make a trade-off among heavy motion capture systems, intrusive athlete equipment, and measurement accuracy. For instance, when using IMUs on limbs, segmental angles (i.e., angle between two limbs) are usually assessed, whereas the heavier motion systems that involve full-body markers allow building an anthropometric model to assess joint angles (Guignard, Rouard, Chollet, & Seifert, 2017b). This latter system is more accurate as it provides the exact centre of rotation of the joint but it is more intrusive for the athletes. Therefore, scientists and practitioners must always deal with the representativeness of the task design, the measurement accuracy, the limitations of the data collection setting, and the complexity and time consumption of the post-processing (i.e., data analysis) for providing feedback to the practitioners and stakeholders.

In short, to design a representative task for collecting data during the training session, practitioners need to design tasks that consider interacting constraints on movement behaviours (i.e., action fidelity/realism), adequately sample informational variables from the specific performance environments (i.e., relevant affordances), and ensure the functional coupling between perception and action processes, where progression towards task goal is evident (Araújo & Davids, 2015). Moreover, the technology for data collection and the computational methods for data analysis need to be meaningful for the practitioners. To enhance representative design, tasks should be viewed as: (i) complex and (ii) dynamic, to provide learners with opportunities to explore a variety of task solutions that evolve over time; (iii) novel and related to achievable goals; (iv) supportive of active perception; and (v) providing sufficient access to key sources of information in the surrounding environment (Davids, Araújo, Hristovski, Passos, & Chow, 2012). With these aspects in mind, the present chapter reviews the different design methodologies for data collection, defining the task, the procedures, and relevant technology, with emphasis on reliability (homogeneity or consistency between two systems; stability or reproducibility between test-retest, for instance, inter- and intra-observer equivalence). When reliability is considered, accuracy and precision could be assessed. Accuracy relates to the difference between the measurement and the part's actual value, while precision describes the variation when the same part is measured repeatedly with the same device. Finally, we also look for the validity (degree to which the equipment or capture systems measure what they are theoretically expected to measure) of the different technological devices.

Design Methodologies for Data Collection

Notational Analysis from Video-Based Systems

Notational Analysis Principles

Notational analysis from video-based systems is vastly used for performance analysis in sport. It represents a convenient, practical, and inexpensive procedure for providing information to practitioners by noting and quantifying the recorded performance. The applications of notation and rating have been developed for tactical evaluation, for technical evaluation, for analysis of movement patterns and coordination, with the consequent design of databases and modelling, and for the educational use with both practitioners and players (Hughes & Franks, 2008). The observational rating of athlete performance corresponds to coding (i.e., pattern detection) and sequencing (i.e., timing identification) by an observer. Thanks to advanced software packages (e.g., Dartfish© www.dartfish.com, Hudl Sportscode© www.hudl.com/products/sportscode, Longomatch© www.longomatch.com, nacsport© www.nacsport.com), coding and sequencing are now easier and faster than ever, replacing the fully manual rating techniques of the past. The software allows the direct connection of the video camera with the laptop for live analysis, or importing video clips and mixing several viewing angles for post-competition analysis. The software enables us to create windows and buttons in order to define performance indicators, movement patterns, and action categories that could be quickly identified and coded during live analysis. However, post-competition analysis is also possible, by scrutinizing the game/race (e.g., zoom, slow motion, export of video clip containing notation to provide feedback), which would increase the reliability of the analysis (Hughes & Franks, 2004).

Validity and Reliability of Notational Analysis

A potential limitation of notational analysis is the validity and the reliability of the data collection and analysis, and the ability of the observer(s) to reproduce the coding and sequencing when the assessment is repeated over time.

The validity of notational analysis relates to the degree to which the observation of the human observer measures and quantifies the concept that it is expected to measure and quantify. The reliability of a system corresponds to the equivalence of sets of items from the same test or/and the same method to collect and analyse the data. The reliability is estimated by computing the intra-observer (e.g., by comparing test-retest) and inter-observer equivalence (Hughes & Franks, 2008). Intra- and inter-observer equivalence is crucial to assess the reliability of notational analysis methods, especially when coding and sequencing could be prone to errors. Those errors could come from (i) the number of items to be observed simultaneously (Roberts, Trewartha, & Stokes, 2006), (ii) the clarity of the criteria to identify the beginning/end of the event, (iii) the overlap of several items, and (iv) the conceptual clarity of the items (i.e., performance indicators).

The items to be observed need to be similarly understood by all the observers. Therefore, the reliability of the process also varies depending on how many observers are used, their experience, and the quality of the viewing (which relates to the quality of the video clip) (Hughes & Franks, 2004, 2008). Those errors would lead to large variations of the time taken, the frequency of item observation, or the identification of number and type of events (i.e., athletes movement patterns and team actions) among observers or among several analyses of the same observer (Barris & Button, 2008).

According to Hughes and Franks (2008), applying a test of intra- or inter-observer differences about the mean or median is not enough, and a measure of absolute differences of the means or medians should also be applied. Thus, simple percentage calculation gives the best indicator of reliability, but Hughes and Franks (2008) give recommendations to avoid errors and confusion. Notably, the data should initially retain its sequence and be cross-checked item by item. Reliability tests should be performed on each set of data instead of mean. Careful definition of the variables involved in the percentage calculation is necessary to prevent any error of the reliability study. Given that, Hughes and Franks (2008) advised to compute the percentage differences based upon: $(\Sigma \,(\mathrm{mod}\,(V_1 - V_2)) \,/\, V_{\mathrm{mean}}) \times 100\%$, where V_1 and V_2 are variables, V_{mean} is their mean, mod is modulus, and Σ means 'sum of', which is used to calculate the percentage error for each variable involved in the observation system.

Examples of Studies Looking at Validity and/or Reliability of Notational Analysis

Duthie, Pyne, and Hooper (2003) analysed the reliability of video-based time-motion analysis with ten rugby union players who were individually assessed during 12 competitions by a single observer on two occasions (one month apart). The test-retest reliability was quantified as the typical error of measurement (TEM) and was computed as the standard deviation of the difference score between repeated analysis, divided by $\sqrt{2}$ (Hopkins, 2000), and rated as good (<5%), moderate (5%–9.9%), or poor (>10%) (McInnes, Carlson, Jones, & McKenna, 1995). The total time spent in the movement categories (walking, jogging, striding, sprinting, static exertion, and being stationary) had moderate to poor reliability (5.8%–11.1% TEM). The frequency of individual movements had good to poor reliability (4.3%–13.6% TEM), while the mean duration of individual movements had moderate reliability (7.1%–9.3% TEM). Duthie et al. (2003) concluded that video-based time-motion analysis of rugby players' movements is moderately reliable, with variation in the reliability of different movement categories, where the analysis of jogging had the best reliability and the analysis of stationary and higher intensity activities such as striding and sprinting had the lower reliability. The lower reliability of sprinting analysis may be attributed to differences in the movement patterns between sports, confirming that observers experience might influence their assessment.

This study suggests that individual observers should quantify their reliability when performing time-motion analysis, notably against other systems such as global positioning system (GPS) (Dogramac, Watsford, & Murphy, 2011), inertial measurement unit (IMU) (Dadashi et al., 2013), or video tracking system (Roberts et al., 2006). As an example, Roberts et al. (2006) used a five-camera tracking system to record the distances and running speeds during seven activities (standing, walking, jogging, medium-, high-, maximal-intensity running) in rugby and compared this system to notational analysis. Reliability for both intra- and inter-observer results was measured using typical error of measurement (TEM). For a 20-minute period, the mean distance travelled was $1{,}554 \pm 329$ m and $1{,}446 \pm 163$ m, and the mean number of changes in activity was 184 ± 24 and 458 ± 48 for both the notational and digitizing methods, respectively; mean speeds were greater with a mean absolute difference of $0.13 \ \mathrm{m \cdot s^{-1}}$ in the notational method. Roberts et al. (2006) suggested that using seven items to classify the activity might increase the difficulty of the selection of the appropriate activity during the notational analysis. Moreover, the video tracking system allowed informing on deceleration/acceleration during activity whereas notational analysis only provided mean speeds. As a consequence, the reliability of the data analysis really depends on the task design and the procedures (e.g., number of observed items to classify activity).

To increase the validity and the reliability, observers can train together to agree on the observed performance indicators, perform blind observations (i.e., without knowing the outcome of other observers), and then make comparisons among their respective analyses, to discuss any gaps among their observations to understand and correct the sources of error, and finally to repeat this process until reaching a high level of reliability. In swimming, Seifert et al. (2006) compared the ability of novice and expert observers to detect the key points defining the arm stroke phases (i.e., entry, glide, catch, pull, push, and recovery). Group comparison of the mean (*t*-test) and of the variance (*F*-test) revealed significant differences for the detection of the catch key point defining the beginning of the pull phase. Additional investigation showed that the training of 50 hours was necessary for novice observers to provide reliable observations. When the observers have a high expertise in observing specific events, non-significant differences were found between the notational analysis data and that of 3D kinematic tracking software (Seifert et al., 2006). Similar results of arm stroke phases and of index of coordination were obtained when notational analyses of expert observers were compared against data computed from IMU (inertial measurement unit composed of 3D accelerometer and 3D gyroscope) (Dadashi et al., 2013). Indeed, a difference of $0.2 \pm 3.9\%$ appeared between the notational analysis from a video-based system and the IMU, which was similar to the inter-observer difference ($1.1 \pm 3.6\%$).

In conclusion, the degree of reliability of notational analysis from a video-based system is not better nor worse than other systems, as it can reveal high reliability when methodological considerations are studied in designing the assessment task and related procedures, in setting the technology device and collecting the data, and in coding and sequencing the data. Notational analysis enables the assessment of kinematic (e.g., movement patterns) and physiological indicators (e.g., type of activity) but only by considering mean values (e.g., mean time for an event or a distance allowing to compute mean speed). Thus, it cannot provide deceleration/acceleration or the intensity of the activity for which the beginning and the end of the event are difficult to assess accurately. Lastly, the number of items, the complexity of these items, the experience of the observers, the temporal constraints to assess the items (e.g., live observation), and the quality of video footage really impact on the reliability of the analysis. Because of the complexity to assess compound metrics such as interpersonal coordination, notational analysis should focus on direct metrics to guarantee the validity and reliability of their measurements (Vilar, Araújo, Davids, & Button, 2012). Therefore, assuming that notational analysis from a video-based system represents a convenient, practical, and inexpensive procedure, the representativeness of the task and the quality of the procedures should be of primarily interest to guarantee a valuable feedback to practitioners and a transferable outcome to the game/race.

2D and 3D Automatic Tracking from Video and Optokinetic Multi-Camera Systems

The great advantage of automatic motion tracking systems is the possibility of continuously tracking athlete(s) without human supervision. Different camera systems such as TV broadcasting, multi-video camera systems, and optokinetic multi-camera systems (Vicon© www.vicon.com, Qualisys© www.qualisys.com, Optitrack© www.optitrack.com) allow 2D or 3D tracking of athletes, using marker or markerless motion capture techniques.

TV Broadcast Tracking Technology

Automated broadcast tracking represents a huge leap forward as it enables us to track the ball and players during 40%–60% of the time of an official football game from a standard television broadcast without the need of additional equipment in stadiums nor the supervision of a human operator (Mortensen & Bornn, 2020; SkillCorner, 2020, www.skillcorner.com). Player's position is obtained from the main broadcast camera using a dynamic pitch calibration, which is applied to the main broadcast camera during its left and right travelling across the football pitch. Tracking data is generated whenever the main camera is used; however; the data generation is not continuous because some players are out of the field of the camera. Therefore, positional data cannot be provided when the broadcast director switches to a player close-up or shows replays. To fill up missing data, extrapolation is done, following a validation study based on a gold standard video multi-camera tracking system (Mortensen & Bornn, 2020; SkillCorner, 2020, www.skillcorner.com).

From a technological perspective, collecting tracking data from the broadcast video in football is the combination of five steps:

i   *View segmentation*: does the main camera capture the current frame or is it from a replay or a close-up view camera?
ii *Detection of the players, the referees, and the ball*: detecting and classifying in each frame.
iii *Homography estimation*: estimating the parameter of the camera to be able to project the detection of the object from the image to their Cartesian coordinates on the football pitch.
iv *Tracking the players, the referees, and the ball*: adding temporal information to track the detection from one frame to the next sequential frame.
v   *Recognition of the players*: identifying the individual players in each frame.

Thus, TV broadcast tracking solves several challenging problems (SkillCorner, 2020):

i   *Homography estimation* in a wide range of stadium sizes without any prior information on the position of the cameras.
ii *Tracking the ball in 3D* (x, y, and z coordinates) at any time of the match. The broadcast feed only includes one camera at a given time, so this estimation needs to be done from a single point of view – traditional triangulation cannot be performed.
iii *Unsupervised player recognition*: player's recognition is not trained with the match prior to the match, but the algorithm is able to recognize a player who was never detected before. This recognition of players during their first match, even when they change to a new jersey, ensures scalability of the product.

iv *Real-time delivery*: video processing is performed at ten frames per second, in real time, with a delay of 2 s on the TV feed – meaning the data is delivered to the practitioners 2 s after the video is received.

Given that all the players are visible only 40%–60% of the match duration, extrapolation of the data must be done. For example, Mortensen and Bornn (2020) extrapolated the data to make prediction about the different activity metrics (i.e., total covered distance, distance at high speed, distance at very high speed, speed < 3.5 $\mathrm{m \cdot s^{-1}}$, 3.5 $\mathrm{m \cdot s^{-1}}$ < speed < 5.7 $\mathrm{m \cdot s^{-1}}$, speed > 5.7 $\mathrm{m \cdot s^{-1}}$, total acceleration, acceleration density, 0.65 $\mathrm{m \cdot s^{-2}}$ < acceleration < 1.46 $\mathrm{m \cdot s^{-2}}$, 1.46 $\mathrm{m \cdot s^{-2}}$ < acceleration < 2.77 $\mathrm{m \cdot s^{-2}}$, acceleration > 2.77 $\mathrm{m \cdot s^{-2}}$) of the players during the unobserved time. The authors based their analysis on 18 home games played by Chelsea FC in the 2014–2015 English Premier League, which included information of 248 players (Mortensen & Bornn, 2020). The authors assessed the reliability of their prediction by computing root mean square predictive error (RMSPE), which is defined as $\mathrm{RMSPE} = \sqrt{\sum(y_i - Y_i)^2/n}$, where Y_i is the predicted value for observation y_i and n is the number of observations, and the coefficient of variation (CV). The CV informs on how large the errors are relative to the values themselves, giving an indication of how much the overall variance in the data was reduced by the given model. Globally, RMSPE and CV values show that the predictions for the various metrics are very accurate. Some of the stratified metrics, i.e., speed >5.7 $\mathrm{m \cdot s^{-1}}$ and very high speed distance, have larger CV values due to the small amount of time players spend in these states, but the RMSPE in these cases was still low enough for use in a practical setting. In particular, the RMSPE for speed >5.7 $\mathrm{m \cdot s^{-1}}$ was still only 6.4 s; for the total distance, the RMSPE was 183 m considering that players travelled on average 3,524 m in each game (Mortensen & Bornn, 2020).

In conclusion, the current state of art concerning TV broadcast tracking is promising as it enables us to predict activities of the players; however, it is not used yet to assess interpersonal coordination or any other metrics relative to the collective behaviour of the team. It presents an advantage for improving online match analysis. Moreover, one can believe that similar techniques can be used for training session analysis. However, during practice, the camera setting could be better controlled to avoid unobserved players and spatial occlusion.

Multi-Video Camera Systems

When using a multi-video camera system, including different perspectives and possible wide lens, parallax and distortion (translation and rotation) must be corrected in reference to calibrated plan (for 2D analysis) or volume (for 3D analysis) using enough point of calibration (like a grid or chessboard for a plan). Coordinate reconstruction, made by direct linear transformation (DLT) (Abdel-Aziz & Karara, 1971), would be improved when using more calibration points in each field of view (Brewin & Kerwin, 2003). Any error in the camera-calibration process primarily introduces a systematic error in the following data processing. Another source of error is the digitizing process. Indeed, the simple manual digitization of anatomical landmarks is error-prone and intra- and inter-operator reliability of the digitizing process must be computed, as previously described for notational analysis. In order to reduce the error of calibration and the error of digitizing, it is recommended to record the volume in which the task takes place with enough cameras, as the tracking accuracy is dependent on the number of cameras. However, a high number of cameras also increase the demand of the digitizing process, especially in the case of manual or semi-automatic tracking. Manual digitization is always very long and is a major issue of manual video tracking (Mooney et al., 2015; Wilson et al., 1999). For instance, according to Psycharakis and Sanders (2008), it took 27 hours to digitize four-stroke cycles in swimming. Therefore, automatic tracking is a major advancement. Such automatic tracking is based on pattern recognition using various types of algorithms (based on colour, shape, motion, etc.) to track an object or an area containing several objects, with respective limitations to each algorithm. For instance, non-linear displacement of the object and spatial occlusion might be an issue when using an algorithm based on motion or trajectory recognition. Ambient light might be an issue when using an algorithm based on colour recognition. As an example, water clarity and light reflection, parallax effect at the water-air interface (Kwon, 1999), distortion problems and pixel contrast between the swimmer and the background (Ichikawa, Ohgi, & Miyaji, 1998), and turbulence or bubble formation (Mooney et al., 2015) are all factors that hamper continuity in the recorded data. Due to these complications of kinematic measurements in water, an increase in error reconstruction occurs up to 42% compared with similar on-land analyses (Silvatti et al., 2013). To overcome issues due to temporary occlusion, blurry image, or any other problems responsible of missing or poor data, automatic tracking algorithms should integrate temporal information to consider a sequence of images (e.g., moving window, block matching) instead of conducting a frame-by-frame analysis for which filling the gaps due to missing data might be an issue (e.g., Al Alwani & Chahir, 2016; Benezeth, Jodoin, Saligrama, & Rosenberger, 2009; Bouziane, Chahir, Molina, & Jouen, 2013; Chahir, Djerioui, Brik, & Ladjal, 2019; Lassoued, Zagrouba, & Chahir, 2016; Liang, Chahir, Molina, Tijus, & Jouen 2014).

Finally, instead of tracking a particular object or body markers, for which marker occlusion could be an issue, one approach consists of using markerless 3D motion capture systems (Mündermann, Corazza, & Andriacchi, 2006), using deep learning-based approaches with 2D or 3D pose estimation (Iskakov, Burkov, Lempitsky, & Malkov, 2019; Pavlakos, Zhou, & Daniilidis, 2018; Pavllo, Feichtenhofer, Grangier, & Auli, 2019) or RGB-depth cameras such as Microsoft Kinect™ (Clark et al., 2012; Gao, Yu, Zhou, & Du, 2015; Liddy et al., 2017; Pfister, West, Bronner, & Noah, 2014; Schmitz, Ye, Shapiro,

Yang, & Noehren, 2014). Liddy et al. (2017) investigated the temporal shift between the Microsoft Kinect^{TM} system and the optokinetic Vicon system during a bi-manual coordination task at frequencies ranging between 1 and 3.33 Hz. They observed that the highest motion frequencies generated the lowest temporal shifts between the two systems, but the authors demonstrated a reduction in the structural differences in the hand trajectories with an increase in frequency. Regarding pose estimation, OpenPose (Cao, Hidalgo, Simon, Wei, & Sheikh, 2018; Nakano et al., 2020) is a popular open-source pose estimation technology that could be used as a 3D markerless motion capture technique. In three different tasks (walking, countermovement jumping, and ball throwing), Nakano et al. (2020) examined the accuracy (by computing the mean absolute error – MAE) of 3D markerless motion capture technique, using OpenPose with multiple synchronized video cameras in comparison with optical marker-based motion capture. The results indicated that 47% of the MAEs were <20 mm, 80% were <30 mm, and 10% were >40 mm. The primary reason for mean absolute errors exceeding 40 mm was that OpenPose failed to track the participant's pose in 2D images owing to failures, such as recognition of an object as a human body segment or replacing one segment with another depending on the image of each frame. Therefore, the authors concluded that OpenPose-based markerless motion capture can be used for human movement science with an accuracy of 30 mm or less. Advanced algorithms for 3D reconstruction (e.g., patch-based multi-view stereo – PMVS, Furukawa & Ponce, 2010; Poisson surface reconstruction – PSR, Kazhdan, Bolitho & Hoppe, 2006) and for pose estimation (e.g., iterative closest point – ICP, Sandau et al., 2014) allow very accurate 3D markerless motion capture. For instance, using those algorithms, Sandau et al. (2014) assessed the 3D joint rotations in the lower extremities and obtained good reliability between markerless and marker motion capture systems for ankle and hip flexion/extension angles as well as for hip abduction/adduction (mean of difference < 1°, root mean square deviation < 3°). However, the hip and knee internal/external rotations, knee abduction/adduction, and ankle inversion/eversion were less reliable (Sandau et al., 2014). In conclusion, gold standard is still tracking motion capture of body markers, as also done with optokinetic systems. However, progress in computer vision, and machine and deep learning techniques offers promising, quick, and inexpensive 2D and 3D markerless motion tracking from single or multi-camera system, which does not require equipment to be placed on the athletes and favours data collection in the ecological context of performance.

Optokinetic Camera Systems

Three-dimensional (3D) optokinetic analyses are based on the automatic detection of reflective markers positioned on joints and are currently the gold standard for motion capture. These systems require the use of multiple cameras, for which the setup, position, resolution, and calibration determine a volume within which movement is analysed. Ambient light should be controlled to guarantee a good tracking of the reflective body markers, which makes opto-kinetic camera systems more suitable for indoor data collection than outside. Tracking issues depend on the number of tracked objects, the degree of the spatial and temporal occlusion between objects, the specification of the camera (e.g., resolution 5–26 MP, frame rate 100–1,400 Hz, narrow to wide lens, maximum capture distance 10–40 m), the number of cameras, and the captured distance and volume in which object(s) are tracked (Barris & Button, 2008; Pers, Bon, Kovacic, Sibila, & Dezman, 2002). As for multi-video camera systems, this volume is therefore dependent on the number of cameras used for measurement, which is proportional to the accuracy of the spatial-temporal recordings (de Jesus et al., 2015). However, the more the cameras used, the higher the cost of the optokinetic system (Carse, Meadows, Bowers, & Rowe, 2013). This financial limitation was addressed with the emergence of affordable 3D motion analysis systems (e.g., OptiTrack system) that provide accurate solutions to track reflective markers (Carse et al., 2013; Thewlis, Bishop, Daniell, & Paul, 2013). Indeed, Thewlis et al. (2013) found an absolute angular difference between the Vicon system and the OptiTrack system that did not exceed 4.2° during gait. With the same systems, Carse et al. (2013) also identified a high degree of agreement in the recorded mean vector magnitudes (1–3 mm) when distances between markers were compared. Although cost is no longer a direct limitation to the use of 3D optokinetic systems, they tend to be used mostly in laboratory conditions (Ceccon et al., 2013). Indeed, it is still constraining and time-consuming to transport and set up these devices in ecological contexts of performance, to finally obtain measurements in a restricted volume of analysis. For instance, optokinetic camera systems could only characterize three to four cycles in swimming, whereas swimmers performed three times more cycles in a 25-m lap. Although gold standard optokinetic camera systems are accurate, they fail to provide easy and rapid measurement of multiple cycles through an event, and more globally the volume of the data collection is a limitation that makes their utilization difficult to track an area as large as a football pitch.

Sensors

Wearable sensors were developed to compensate the lack of portability of multi-camera systems (both multi-video cameras and optokinetic systems), as they are wireless, small, and light. A second limitation of multi-camera systems relates to the lack of control of the ambient environment in which data are collected (in terms of light, calibration volume, and/or area, etc.) which led scientists to develop new devices to track the behavioural dynamics over long periods of time, involving time-series analysis. Indeed, getting 10%–20% of an event cannot represent the performance during a whole event; therefore, new technologies are requested to track athletes' behaviours over a longer period of time, covering all the area or volume of performance. To overcome the previous limitations, devices such as smartwatches, smartphones, global positioning system (GPS), inertial measurement unit (IMU), or eye tracking system (glasses) have been developed. Those devices are often of low cost, light, user-centric, portable (i.e., wearable), and hence easy to use in field conditions, which could favour *in situ* and representative design of the task and procedures. In comparison to 3D multi-cameras systems, smartwatches, GPS, and IMUs can record a high volume of continuous data over an entire competitive or training event.

Smartwatch, Smartphone, and Global Positioning System (GPS)

In regard to smartwatches, Mooney et al. (2017) have tested the reliability of two commercially swimming activity monitors (Finis *Swimsense*® and Garmin *Swim*™) against a multi-video camera system used for notational analysis. Ten swimmers had to swim 1,500 m in the four swimming techniques, then the reliability of the smartwatches was assessed for five features (i.e., stroke swimming technique, swim distance, lap time, stroke count, and average speed). High reliability was found to detect the swimming technique, the swim distance, and the number of swimming laps performed in the middle of a swimming interval; however, the number of laps performed at the beginning and end of an interval were not as accurately timed. In addition, a statistical difference was found for stroke count measurements, which affect the accuracy of stroke rate, stroke length, and average speed measurements. Mooney et al. (2017) concluded that these smartwatches appear suited for recreational use, but further development to improve accuracy of the lap time and stroke count detection would be required for competitive settings. In running, Pobiruchin, Suleder, Zowalla, and Wiesner (2017) used a pre-race and post-race survey to investigate the accuracy of tracked distances recorded by smart devices (e.g., smartwatches and smartphones). The mean of the track distances recorded by mobile phones with combined application (mean absolute error of 0.35 km) was significantly different to GPS-enabled sport watches (mean absolute error of 0.12 km) for the half-marathon event. Again, smart devices appear suitable for recreational use but not for scientific purpose.

The GPS integrated in a smart suit or in a bra is regularly used to quantify the external load in team sports (Cummins, Orr, O'Connor, & West, 2013; Hausler, Halaki, & Orr, 2016; Jennings, Cormack, Coutts, Boyd, & Aughey, 2010; Johnston et al., 2012; Scott, Scott, & Kelly, 2016; Willmott, James, Bliss, Leftwich, & Maxwell, 2019). Scott et al. (2016) investigated the reliability of GPS in a team sport setting, with a particular focus on measurements of distance, speed, and accelerations across sampling rates of 1, 5, 10, and 15 Hz GPS. Low sampling rate GPS (1 and 5 Hz) exhibited limitations in measuring distance during high-intensity running, speed and short linear running (particularly those involving changes of direction), whereas high sampling rate GPS (10 and 15 Hz) appeared more reliable across linear and team sport simulated running (Scott et al., 2016). Several studies confirmed the higher validity and reliability of GPS with high sample rate for distance and speed measurements in team sports, especially for low-to-moderate speeds (below 20 $km \cdot h^{-1}$) (Gray, Jenkins, & Andrews, 2010; Jennings et al., 2010; Johnston et al., 2012; Waldron, Worsfold, Twist, & Lamb, 2011). For instance, Jennings et al. (2010) observed a lower coefficient of variation (1.4%–2.6%) during walking for a 5 Hz GPS than during sprinting over a 20-m distance (19.7%–30%). Similarly, these authors observed higher coefficients of variation for the same activity (30.8% during walking and 77.2% during sprinting) over a 10-m distance with a 1 Hz GPS (Jennings et al., 2010). Finally, as already mentioned by Scott et al. (2016), the reliability of GPS is also affected by tight change of direction as Jennings et al. (2010) observed a lower coefficient of variation for gradual (11.5%) than for tight (15.2%) change of direction during walking. Therefore, assuming that speed measurement is prone to error at high speed (above 20 $km \cdot h^{-1}$) and during non-linear run with tight changes of direction, cautions might be considered when practitioners break players' activity into speed zones between 0 and 36 $km \cdot h^{-1}$ (Cummins et al., 2013). When such breaks are made, possible differences in the number of sprints at high intensity or in the time spent in high-speed zone due to gender, player's position in the field (attackers/defenders), or age may hide lack of reliability. In fact, few studies assessed the reliability of GPS against gold standard motion capture system (Randers et al., 2010; Waldron et al., 2011).

Randers et al. (2010) compared the activity of 20 football players during a match using four different motion capture systems (a video-based time-motion analysis system – VTM, a semi-automatic multiple-camera system – MCS, and two commercially available GPS systems: 5 Hz GPS and 1 Hz GPS). Although those four systems were able to track the players, significant differences in the total distance covered during the match were observed between the GPS (10.72 ± 0.70 km for the 5 Hz GPS and 9.52 ± 0.89 km for the 1 Hz GPS) and the other two systems (10.83 ± 0.77 km for the MCS and 9.51 ± 0.74 km for the VTM). The distance covered by high-intensity running was significantly different between 5 Hz GPS (2.03 ± 0.60 km) and MCS (2.65 ± 0.53 km), and between 1 Hz GPS (1.66 ± 0.44 km) and both MCS (2.65 ± 0.53 km) and VTM (1.61 ± 0.37 km). The distance covered by sprinting was significantly different between 1 Hz GPS (0.23 ± 0.16 km) and both VTM (0.38 + 0.18 km) and MCS (0.42 ± 0.17 km), whereas 5 Hz GPS (0.37 ± 0.19 km) did not significantly differ with the VTM and MCS. Randers et al. (2010) concluded that there were large between-system differences in the identification of the absolute distances covered, implying that any comparison of results using different match analysis systems should be done with caution.

In another study, Waldron et al. (2011) investigated the validity and reliability of a 5 Hz GPS and timing gates (Brower Timing Systems, Draper, UT) to measure sprinting speed and distance in rugby players, and the reliability of proper accelerations recorded via GPS–accelerometer integration. Results of validity indicated that the GPS measurements systematically underestimated both distance and timing gate speed (coefficient of variation ranged between 4.81% and 9.81%). When the GPS measurements were compared between two tests, a high reliability was observed for all variables of distance and speed (coefficient of variation ranged between 1.62% and 2.3%). However, the timing gates were more reliable (coefficient of variation ranged between 1% and 1.54%) than equivalent GPS measurements. Finally, acceleration measurements (via GPS–accelerometer integration) were less reliable (coefficient of variation ranged between 4.69% and 14.12% when peak acceleration and frequency are compared between two tests). Waldron et al. (2011) concluded that the timing gates and the GPS were reliable systems to assess speed and distance, although the validity of the GPS remains questionable. The error found in acceleration measurements (via GPS–accelerometer integration) indicates the limits of this device for detecting changes in performance. One way to improve the accuracy of the GPS could be by fuzzing data from GPS, IMU, camera, and digital map (Baranski & Strumillo, 2012). Baranski and Strumillo (2012) did so in pedestrian navigation, for 90% of the navigation time, and the algorithm was able to estimate a pedestrian location with an error smaller than 2 m, compared to an error of 6.5 m for a navigation based solely on GPS (Baranski & Strumillo, 2012). In conclusion, advanced sensor fuzzing GPS, accelerometer, and local radio system might offer promising perspectives to improve the measurement reliability for distance and speed. According to the reliability of GPS measurement, multi-camera motion capture systems seem preferred to track players' location in the field and then assess advanced metrics such as interpersonal coordination within and between teams.

Inertial Measurement Unit (IMU)

Generally, IMUs are composed of various sensors such as an accelerometer, gyroscope, and magnetometer, which offer a wide range of measurement opportunities. Notably, the signal of these sensors can be fuzzed to investigate the IMU orientation in external 3D reference (e.g., Earth reference defined by gravity, east and south), which is useful to compute angles. IMUs could be used to provide low-level metrics (e.g., distance, type of activity, stride frequency, and stride length) and high-level metrics (e.g., Euler angles, rotation matrix, quaternion, used to assess segmental and joint angles, and then coordination between joints/limbs; Poitras et al., 2019; Sabatini, 2011; Seel, Raisch, & Schauer, 2014). Moreover, as mentioned previously, IMUs could record data over a long period and then discrete features can be extracted, or in the case of cyclic activities (e.g., rowing, cycling, swimming, running) time-series analysis can be conducted such as inter-cyclic variability investigation. As an example in swimming, Dadashi, Millet, and Aminian (2016) analysed movement and coordination patterns over more than 5,000 cycles during a 400 m front crawl.

Although IMUs have undergone rapid development, the computation of high-level metrics such as joint or segmental angles that are based on the computation of segment rotations remains error-prone and requires step-by-step approach (e.g., IMU positioning on the body, calibration, data collection, and post-processing) to obtain accurate and valid metrics. According to the studies of Teufl, Miezal, Taetz, Fröhlich, and Bleser (2018) in a walking task and Ahmadi, Rowlands, and James (2010) in the tennis serve task, positioning IMUs on rigid clusters rather than directly onto the skin of the participants should provide more accurate results. Indeed, such estimations of the 3D error surface motion of the cluster due to limb movement should be subtracted from the calculated angles to minimize the error due to marker movements (Ahmadi et al., 2010). Thus, both static and dynamic calibration procedures are required to compute accurate angles or reduce offsets (Seel et al., 2014) due to sensor movements during the recordings. Calibrations enable us to synchronize all the IMUs, and to express their positions in the bone anatomical frame (a 3D coordinate transformation to an absolute system of coordinates; Dadashi, Crettenand, Millet, & Aminian, 2012). Such a frame change (from IMU reference to Earth reference) enables the extraction of the gravity vector (Earth's attraction) on the sensor acceleration (Seel et al., 2014). In addition, Fantozzi et al. (2016) advised that calibration should be performed again in the middle of a testing if the operators suspect possible movements of the IMU on the limb. Nevertheless, the accuracy of such calibrations is still dependent on the accuracy with which the athlete performs calibration procedures (Seel et al., 2014). Therefore, Seel et al. (2014) proposed a method to cope with the possible misalignment of the IMU and the limbs by using arbitrary knee motions during the calibration process. With arbitrary knee motions of 10 seconds, these authors computed unit-length direction vectors that were dependent on the initial position of the IMU on the limb. Then, Seel et al. (2014) integrated the difference of the angular rates around the joint axis during flexion-extension motion, which yielded a highly accurate but slowly drifting joint angle. This angle was combined in a sensor fusion with a noisy but drift-less joint angle estimate that was calculated from the measured accelerations (Seel et al., 2014). In comparison to optokinetic Vicon system, their model provided valid results for knee joint estimation during six gait trials, with mean RMSE values of 3.30°.

After calibration issue, another issue relates to the progressive drift in the gyroscope measurements with time. Indeed, for any type of measurement (i.e., static, simple 2D, or complex 3D recordings), drift accumulates due to noise or small offsets in the measurement of angular velocity (Zhou & Hu, 2010). Moreover, although IMU orientation can be computed by time integration of the gyroscope recordings, this process reveals the low-frequency gyro bias drift (Sabatini, 2011). In order to limit this phenomenon, the inclination of the IMU can be estimated from the accelerometer, which is drift-free and combines its measurements with the gravity vector. From there, the combination of the recordings of both sensors may become a viable solution to correct the gyroscope's drift and better estimate the 3D sensor position. Zhou and Hu (2010) used a Kalman filter that compares inclinations measured from the accelerometers and gyroscopes, and the difference between them is then used to correct the estimated orientation. They also integrated the segment lengths to better estimate the displacements of each segment (Zhou & Hu, 2010; Zhou, Stone, Hu, & Harris, 2008). In swimming, Seifert, Komar, Hérault, and Chollet (2014), and Dadashi et al. (2012) observed such a drift for angle computation and velocity assessment, respectively. Seifert, Komar, Hérault, and Chollet (2014) proposed a simple correction of this (pseudo-linear) drift on the elbow angle time series by wrapping the peaks and valleys of the signal. This procedure gives peak-and-valley shape-preserving splines (and in some cases lines, when the drift is perfectly linear), which are considered as maximal and minimal values of the recordings. This procedure cannot provide absolute angle values but only relative values that were normalized between −1 and 1, and which allow comparison between cycles of a time series (Seifert, Komar, Hérault, & Chollet, 2014).

Validity, Reliability, and Accuracy of IMU

The validity of IMU could be assessed with Spearman's rank correlation (or Spearman r) to verify the statistical dependence between the values obtained from the IMUs and a gold standard system such as optokinetic multi-camera system. However, such computation ignores measurement bias, which was assessed by Bland and Altman analyses (1986) to better characterize the validity of the IMUs by comparing the agreement between the systems. Limits of agreement (LoA) are computed as mean bias ± 1.96*SD (Bland & Altman, 1986).

Taylor, Miller, and Kaufman (2017) performed a dynamic validation test on a wheel to examine the validity of the IMUs and found that IMUs were more accurate at lower velocities compared with the gold standard. Cutti, Giovanardi, Rocchi, and Davalli (2006) found similar results and emphasized that IMU errors of measurement typically increase with velocity.

Assuming that gyroscopes are prone to drift, the reliability was estimated by computing the internal consistency of the data over time (Dadashi et al., 2012). Therefore, the normalized pairwise variability index ($nPVI$) (Sandnes & Jian, 2004) could be used because it evaluates the spatial variability in cyclical time series (e.g., computation over each period of a sinusoidal signal):

$$nPVI = \left[\frac{\sum_{C_k=1}^{N} \left| \frac{A_{\text{sensors}} - A_{\text{opto}}}{\left(A_{\text{sensors}} + A_{\text{opto}} \right) / 2} \right|}{N} \right] \times 100$$

where C_k is the kth measure performed by both compared systems, and N the total quantity of acquired data by the corresponding materials. Reliability could also be quantified as the time difference between the occurrence of local maximums on the optokinetic signals and that of the IMU signals. For instance, Zanone and Kelso (1992) propose to compute the discrete relative phase between the two signals when they are periodic or pseudo-periodic:

$$\theta = \frac{t_1 - t_2}{T} \times 360$$

with the discrete relative phase computed in degrees; t_1 corresponds to the shifting peak of the IMU signal, t_2 the shifting peak of the optokinetic signal, and T the period of the optokinetic signal. When computing the discrete relative phase, any transitory or recurrent temporal shifting of the IMU signals relative to the gold standard could be quantified.

Finally, the data accuracy could be assessed by computing the root mean square error ($RMSE$) between the whole time series obtained by IMUs and the optokinetic multi-camera system (Rein, 2012):

$$RMSE = \sqrt{\sum_{i=1}^{n} \left(A_{\text{opto}(i)} - A_{\text{sensors}(i)} \right)^2 \Big/ n}$$

with n being the total number of data pairs compared – at the same time i – between the systems. A value of RMSE close to zero indicates a limited dispersion of the data registered by the IMUs relative to the values obtained by an optokinetic multi-camera system. Zhou and Hu (2010), who tested different motion speeds for upper limb movements, did not find any significant impact of speed on RMSE values (absolute mean error around 3°) between optokinetic Qualisys multi-camera system and Xsens suit of IMUs (www. xsens.com). Nüesch, Roos, Pagenstert, and Mündermann (2017) observed RMSE values ranging between 5° and 10° for both IMU knee angular measurements and the gold standard during a walking test. In swimming, de Magalhães et al. (2013, 2015) investigated shoulder kinematics during five si front crawl strokes, measuring angular discrepancies between a stereophotogrammetric system and IMUs. Angles between the upper arm and the thorax revealed RMSE values ranging from 5° to 10° (mean value at 7°). During the same task performed over nearly 20 stroke cycles, Fantozzi et al. (2016) reported mean RMSE values of 7° for both systems, with the largest differences observed for elbow pronation-supination and flexion-extension (10° and 15°, respectively). Following previous research, an error of 2° or less is considered acceptable, as such errors are probably too small to require explicit consideration during data interpretation (Cuesta-Vargas, Galán-Mercant, & Williams, 2010; McGinley, Baker, Wolfe, & Morris, 2009).

Errors of between 2° and 5° are also likely to be regarded as reasonable but may require consideration in data interpretation. Finally, Cuesta-Vargas et al. (2010) suggested that errors above 5° should raise concern and may be large enough to mislead interpretation. These recommendations fit with the recent systematic review by Poitras et al. (2019), who reviewed the research that compared IMUs to motion capture systems for body joint angle estimation. To conclude, IMUs represent a promising way to assess human motion in real time and in ecological context of performance, as it corresponds to wireless, small, and light devices that can record data over a long time. Low-level and high-level metrics could be collected; however, the higher the complexity of the metrics computation, the greater the cautions of the procedures (e.g., position of the IMUs on the body, calibration and settings, synchronization, data processing).

Ecophysical Variables to Capture the Ecological Dynamics of Sport Performance

Sport performance implies an understanding of both how individual abilities match environmental opportunities and how they dynamically interact within the successive tasks of a match or a race. Therefore, the variables of interest cannot ignore the context where performance unfolds. More to the point, the sources of data cannot be solely located in the performer but need to capture how the player is adjusting and achieving the task goals of the performance environment. The role of affordances and the perceptual attunement and readiness to act on them seem to be of paramount importance. This is the concern of the ecological dynamics framework. In particular, ecological dynamics theoretical approach starts from the understanding that (i) performance emerges from the performer-environment system; (ii) to understand the performance of an individual, an analysis of the behaviours offered by his/her environment (i.e., affordances) is necessary; and (iii) performance emerges (as a result of self-organization) under interacting constraints (Araújo & Davids, 2018; Araújo et al., 2020; Button et al., 2020).

This approach implies that ecophysical variables (Araújo et al., 2020) are the best starting point to capture intelligent behaviour (see Chapter 1). These are variables that express the fit between the environment and the performer's adaptations. As mentioned before, environmental properties may directly inform what an individual can and cannot do and this is why representative assessment tasks are so important (Araújo & Davids, 2015; Davids et al., 2012). An important challenge for researchers and practitioners is to capture ecophysical variables predicated on perception-action couplings during continuous, emergent, performer-environment interactions in sports. Next we present examples from research in sport sciences in football, rugby, swimming, and climbing.

Football

Carrilho et al. (2020) captured team synergic properties, using spatiotemporal data from one match of the 2018 FIFA World Cup in Russia, to analyse the ecophysical variable 'player-ball-goal angles' in a cluster phase analysis. Relative phase analysis (RPA) has been used in team sports to measure synchronization (e.g., Travassos, Araújo, Duarte, & McGarry, 2012). RPA is based on the difference of the oscillation between two phases, expressed as a measure of their relative phase angle, defined by their angular frequency (ω) and their initial phase ($\phi0$). Two oscillators in a time series can be locked in an in-phase mode of synchronization, if their angle difference holds near 0° or in an anti-phase, if the angle is near 180°. Based on this idea, cluster phase analysis (CPA) also measures synchronization, but it is based on the relationship among the oscillatory movement of a group of elements, using the Kuramoto order parameter (Duarte et al., 2013). Therefore, differently from RPA, CPA measures synchrony among the oscillating phases of the elements within a group. In the study of Carrilho et al. (2020) they analysed player-ball-goal angles (PBGAs) in CPA to directly measure player-environment relationships and capture the properties of team synergic behaviour (Araújo & Davids, 2016). The ball, the goals, and the players were identified as key ecological variables of the football match, as they inform and constrain the behaviour of players. Therefore, by using the PBGA they capture the link between players and performance environment, providing ecological explanatory value to CPA. The synchronization measures obtained from CPA were a direct result of changes in the PBGA, which continually captured the displacement of the players on the pitch, in relation to the goal and the ball.

Positional data were provided by the Portuguese Football Federation (FPF) and obtained by the TRACAB, Optical Tracking System (Chyron-Hego) (see Linke, Link, & Lames, 2020). The dataset consisted of positional data of every player (n = 28) and the ball (n = 1), captured at 25 Hz with spatial resolution of 0.01 m. For CPA measures, each cluster (team) was constituted by the respective players on the pitch. The PBGA, θ_k, for each player, k, ranged from 0 to π and was calculated at every time frame, t_i, with the vertex on the ball, using the planar coordinates of each player, ball, and goal as represented by Equation (3.1). The PBGAs were calculated as the goal was being attacked.

$$\theta_k(t_i) = a\tan2(\|(\mathbf{P}_k(t_i) - \mathbf{B}(t_i)) \otimes (\mathbf{G}(t_i) - \mathbf{B}(t_i)\|,$$
$$(\mathbf{P}_k(t_i) - \mathbf{B}(t_i)) \cdot (\mathbf{G}(t_i) - \mathbf{B}(t_i))) \tag{3.1}$$

In Equation (3.1), the PBGA, θ_k, was calculated using the planar coordinates for each player, $\mathbf{P}_k$, ball, $\mathbf{B}$, and goal, $\mathbf{G}$, at every time frame, t_i, expressed as vectors (Carrilho et al., 2020).

Results showed that the cluster phase values (synchronization) for the home team increased compared to the away team and that changing the role from with ball to without ball increased synchronization. The player-team relative phase, the player-ball-goal angles relative frequency, and the team configurations showed that variations of synchronization might indicate critical performance changes (ball possession changes, goals scored, etc.). PBGSs coherently captured the properties of team synergic behaviour using the synchrony measures. Moreover, CPA, with the PBGA, may capture changes in performance outcomes, before they happen, expressed in the dynamics of the synchronization values. This study indicated that variations in synchronization showed changes in the equilibrium of the performance of the team, which can be related to changes in performance outcomes. In short, this ecophysical variable (PBGAs) enabled the direct measurement of the player-environment link, as the measures were directly influenced by the positioning of players in relation to key ecological variables.

Rugby

Passos et al. (2008, 2009) identified an ecophysical variable that described space-time relations of attacker-defender dyads in rugby. Attackers were required to run past defenders with the ball starting from a position 10 m from the try line. Ecophysical variable values were calculated based on an angle between the defender-attacker vector and an imaginary horizontal line parallel to the try line, with its origin located in the defender's position. This ecophysical variable revealed an angle close to +90° before the attacker reached the defender's location, and close to 290° after the attacker successfully passed the defender, with a zero crossing point emerging precisely when the attacker passed the defender (Passos et al., 2009). Following this empirical evidence, we modelled this attacker-defender-score line system dynamics (Araújo, Diniz, Passos, & Davids, 2014). Importantly, despite the potentially huge variability of behavioural trajectories that both players might undertake, this system was attracted to one of the three states: defender's tackle, defender's tackle with advantage for the attacker, and attacker's try. The potential function that modelled this rugby system could describe its dynamics because players and environment were captured due to the ecophysical variable.

Swimming

In swimming biomechanics, kinematics of the swimmers is often assessed through a 3D multi-camera system (Bernardina et al., 2016, 2017; de Jesus et al., 2015; Figueiredo, Machado, Vilas-Boas, & Fernandes, 2011; Gourgoulis et al., 2008), in order to identify key points of the stroke cycle (e.g., hand entry into water, catch point, maximal forward coordinate, maximal backward coordinate, and hand exit from the water; Aujouannet, Bonifazi, Hintzy, Vuill-erme, & Rouard, 2006), which enable us to define stroke phases (e.g., outward, inward; propulsive and non-propulsive phases; Chollet, Chalies, & Chatard, 2000; Ribeiro et al., 2017). Usually, these measurements are conducted within an egocentric reference. Thus, hand propulsion is often expressed in relation to the shoulder position and in reference to the centre of mass. It does not mean that egocentric reference is meaningless, but it does not capture how swimmers interact with the aquatic environment, e.g., the water plan of the swimming pool or the swimming axis (Guignard et al., 2017a). According to ecological dynamics framework, ecophysical variables such as the angle between the trunk and the water level, or between the arm and the gravitational direction would indicate when the swimmers are in streamline position and how hydrodynamics is disturbed (e.g., by yow, pitch, and rolling body motion), for instance when breathing or swimming against fluid flow (Guignard et al., 2017a, 2020). For this purpose, Guignard et al. (2017a, 2020) used IMU to assess proximal (between upper arm and arm) and distal (between hand and arm) inter-segmental angles and coordination.

Climbing

Although the essence of climbing relates to outdoors, sport climbing becomes increasingly popular and is performed in climbing gym (i.e., artificial climbing wall), where root setters can design very different climbing problems to provide a rich landscape of affordances that would enable transfer of acquired skills to outside. In order to assess the effect of route design on performance, several ecophysical variables could be measured such as the ratio between the motion time and the stationary time (Orth, Kerr, Davids, & Seifert, 2017; Orth, Davids, Chow, & Brymer, & Seifert, 2018a; Seifert et al., 2018), and more recently Seifert, Hacques, Rivet, and Legreneur (2020) presented a new device (Luxov® Touch, Luxov, Arnas, France, http://www.luxov-connect.com/en/products/) to assess the contact time on each hold, in order to investigate the hold-by-hold fluency. The contact time is an ecophysical variable that allows locating which hold involves longer time spent stationary, which often reflects the 'crux' point (i.e., most difficult section of the route). It gives information to root setters and practitioners to understand how the route design influences the climbing fluency. The lack of fluency could also be investigated by spatial indicators such as the geometric index of entropy that reflects the complexity of the climbing path (Figure 3.1) (Orth, Davids, & Seifert, 2018b; Sibella, Frosio, Schena, & Borghese, 2007; Watts, España-Romero, Ostrowski, & Jensen, 2020) or by the smoothness of the body displacement (jerk movement that corresponds to the derivation of acceleration; Seifert, Orth et al., 2014).

Lastly, Seifert, Boulanger, Orth, and Davids (2015), and Orth and colleagues (2018b) examined how an ecophysical variable that captures the body

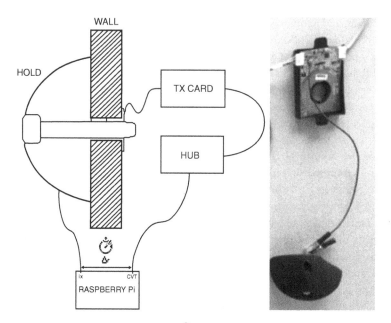

FIGURE 3.1 Instrumented holds Luxov® Touch system.

roll relative to the wall can explain the variation in climbing fluency. For this purpose, the route setter designed three different routes by manipulating the hold orientation and the number of available edges for grasping. A horizontal-edge route was designed to allow horizontal hold grasping when the trunk face to the wall was observed. A vertical-edge route was designed to allow vertical hold grasping, where the more challenging trunk side to the wall usually emerges in experienced climbers. Finally, a double-edge route was designed to invite both horizontal and vertical hold grasping. As a route with only vertical-edge holds was very challenging for novice climbers, the double-edge route would allow safe and functional exploration, as climbers could both exploit their stable patterns (i.e., horizontal hold grasping pattern and trunk face to the wall) associated to fluent motion and explore new behaviours (i.e., vertical hold grasping and trunk side to the wall) often associated with less fluent motion (Seifert et al., 2015).

Conclusion

This chapter explained the representativeness of combining accurate and reliable time-motion kinematical analysis to provide a more comprehensive ecological dynamic understanding of the athletic performance. Then, it discussed design methodologies for data collection, defining the task, the procedures, and relevant technology according to the type of sport (individual and collective).

It highlighted devices and variables that describe sports performance by centring its discussion on low-level kinematic performance indicators and related physiological insights. It also examined the combination of these direct performance indicators into compound metrics and requested cautions to design task, to decide for the relevant technology, to set data collection, and to compute metrics. Following ecological dynamics theoretical framework, we presented ecophysical variables as a means to capture the relevant issues of sport performance, given that performance is defined at the level of performer-environment system. Decision often relates to a compromise between validity, accuracy, reliability, and (i) temporal constraints to set, to collect, to analyse, and to provide feedback to practitioners, and (ii) nature of the task and of the environment in which this task is performed, questioning design representativeness.

4

COMPUTATIONAL METRICS TO INSPECT THE ATHLETIC PERFORMANCE

Introduction

The 'take-home message' from the previous chapters and many other recent works is that the athletic performance is part of a complex dynamic system with an underlying massive amount of data (Davids et al., 2014). Therefore, as with any other complex dynamic system, AI has the potential to unravel patterns of behaviours and interactions between athletes that characterize successful performance in different sports (Beal, Norman, & Ramchurn, 2019). Nonetheless, the analysis of highly complex systems is a challenging task, and while Neural Network (NN) has proven to be one of the most recurrent solutions to tackle them, its successful applicability, as the applicability of any alternative approaches for that matter, highly relies on how these methods are 'fed', i.e., the data provided to them.

Chapter 3 introduced some of the many disruptive technologies used nowadays in sports to extract specific performance indicators, such as kinematic and ecophysical variables, from the athletes. It would only make sense that AI methods would somehow process all the huge volume of data coming from these technologies and provide coaches and sports analysts with better information. Yet, it is not that simple (read about the big data problem discussed in Chapter 1). While the most promising state-of-the-art methods can receive 'raw' variables as inputs and still lead to an interesting outcome (such as deep learning algorithms due to their layered and hierarchical learning architecture), this does not hold for most complex systems, such as sports. The representation of the input data and generalization of the learnt patterns have a crucial impact on the performance of AI approaches: poor data representation is likely to lead to a decreased performance of an advanced deep learning method, while good data representation can lead to a high performance of a traditional machine learning method (Najafabadi et al., 2015).

It is therefore imperative to ensure that the data fed to the different AI approaches, while still reliant on the variables acquired using cameras, wearables, and other technologies, is representative. The process of extracting meaningful representative data, commonly known as features, out of raw data is called feature engineering (Nargesian, Samulowitz, Khurana, Khalil, & Turaga, 2017). Features are measurable properties of the process being observed and, even though they can be set as the original (raw) data (e.g., the velocity of the athlete), those are often computed on top of them. As expected, this is a complex problem as it requires not only strong mathematical expertise but also context-related knowledge, which, in this case, would mean a close collaboration between computer scientists, sport scientists, and other sports-related experts. Furthermore, as the number of simultaneous features that can be processed by AI has expanded so drastically due to technological and scientific advances, additional feature selection strategies are needed to reduce the most irrelevant and redundant variables that might jeopardize the performance of the AI approach.

This chapter introduces and algorithmically delineates several football-related metrics computed based on the performance indicators, or variables, extracted from the technologies presented in Chapter 3, which will be subsequently used as features of the pattern recognition architectures presented in Chapter 5. These computational metrics are 'high level' performance indicators that have been used in panoply of works to capture players' performance, including **individual metrics**, such as the fractional-order coefficient of a player's trajectory, and **group metrics**, including network-related metrics.

Individual Metrics

Many experts agree that, just like in self-organized collective systems found in nature, such as ant colonies and bee hives, the overall performance of a football team is more than the sum of all individuals in that team (Hughes, Franks, & Dancs, 2019). Nevertheless, evaluating how these individual athletes react to training competitive loads, how they interact with one another, how they foster goal-scoring opportunities, among other phenomena, can help the coaching staff in setting new strategies and new combinations between players and even control their recovery, thus preventing overreaching and injuries (Düking, Hotho, Holmberg, Fuss, & Sperlich, 2016; Kellmann, 2010).

Hence, the evaluation of the individual athletic performance has been the most explored topic within the performance analysis literature; on one hand, due to its methodological simplicity when compared to group and network analysis, and, on the other hand, because most approaches lead to an outcome that can be put into practice. For instance, if an individual metric is intended to estimate the energy cost of accelerated and decelerated running of a given athlete, as presented in Osgnach, Poser, Bernardini, Rinaldo, and Di Prampero (2010), then it might provide insights about the metabolic power exerted by such athlete and personalize its training to reach the performance of top-class players.

Nonetheless, although insights can be more clearly and directly with-drawn out of individual metrics, they also lead to a major drawback. Individual metrics are centred on the individual and, therefore, they intend to assess the performance of one athlete regardless of the team. While some individual metrics can still be contextualized (e.g., based on the position in the team formation), they do not take into account the interactions established with other players as group and network metrics do. However, the attributes of a team go beyond the player's individual skills, performance statistics, physical fitness, psychological factors, and injuries (Arnason et al., 2004). For that reason, coaches need to consider a panoply of attributes during the player selection process, which is seen as a complex multi-criteria problem with conflicting objectives (Tavana, Azizi, Azizi, & Behzadian, 2013). The proper selection of players and how it leads to an effective team formation is seen as indispensable for reaching the top ranks (Boon & Sierksma, 2003), which cannot be achieved by considering, separately, the performance of every single player.

Notwithstanding on the above downside, and as previously stated, individual metrics are still essential due to their simplicity (when compared to group and network metrics) and their direct benefit for the athlete, as further explained in the next subsequent sections. Among the many subdomains individual metrics could have been divided into, this book describes the two most predominant subdomains – not only because these metrics can be computed based on data acquired with the technologies mentioned in Chapter 3, but, more importantly, because they provide invaluable information to understand and consequently improve the athletic performance.

Kinematic Measures

Tracking approaches and related technologies have been made available, allowing to collect, at every instant, each player's position on the field (Xu, Orwell, Lowey, & Thirde, 2005), and even their body joint configuration (Shan & Westerhoff, 2005). Such spatio-temporal information is considered of the utmost importance to improve the performance understanding, fostering many kinds of analysis, such as kinematical, technical, and tactical (Bartlett, 2014; Carling, Bloomfield, Nelsen, & Reilly, 2008). Chapter 3 listed some of the most relevant technologies able to track kinematic data, with a particular emphasis on the planar position of players over time, such as wearables (GPS, UWB, RFID, etc.) and video analysis. This section refers to some of the most common metrics computed out of such data, including velocity, distance, and orientation, as well as a few less conventional ones, such as the trajectory entropy and its fractional dynamics.

Velocity

Let the planar position of player i, at a certain instant t, in the field, be defined as $x_i[t] \in R^2$, which can be decomposed in its dimensions – herein simplified to the xy-plane of the football field, i.e., $x_i[t] = (x_i[t], y_i[t])$. The average velocity magnitude between consecutive time steps t can be calculated as follows:

$$v_i[t] = \frac{|x_i[t] - x_i[t-1]|}{\Delta t} = \frac{\sqrt{(x_i[t] - x_i[t-1])^2 + (y_i[t] - y_i[t-1])^2}}{\Delta t} \tag{4.1}$$

where Δt is the time interval, or period, between two consecutive measurements, which is here considered as constant.

Distance

The previous definition of the planar position of player i can also be applied to the distance covered by that player within a specific variation t. Its mathematical formulation can be described as follows:

$$d_i[t] = \Delta t \sum_{k=0}^{t} v_i[t] \tag{4.2}$$

Besides the distance covered by a player, other similar metrics may be contemplated, including the distance between players and the distance to the goal, among others. The association between the average velocity magnitude $v_i[t]$ and the distance covered $d_i[t]$ can empower the analysis of player i train load and provide relevant data to understand and distinguish different activities, such as walking and running.

Orientation

A player's position suffers changes over time that depends on player's tactical position. However, as an absolute feature, it is unclear how relevant it might be unless properly contextualized, namely by considering if it contributes to an offensive or defensive action. Therefore, the orientation of a player can provide an additional source of information if associated with the opponent's goal, contributing towards an understanding of specific actions, such as shots and passes.

Given that $x_G[t] = (x_G[t], y_G[t])$ is the middle line position of the opponent goal, the orientation of player i towards it, $\theta_i[t]$, can be calculated as follows:

$$\theta_i[t] = \left(\delta_i[t] - a\tan 2\left((y_G[t] - y_i[t]),\ (x_G[t] - x_i[t]) \right) \right) \tag{4.3}$$

where $\delta_i[t]$ is the angular position of the player i in the field.

Trajectory Entropy

Studying the variability of football players lays the foundations for a whole series of possible new performance analysis methods (Carling, Bradley, McCall, & Dupont, 2016; Couceiro, Clemente, Martins, & Machado, 2014). Some non-linear methods, such as Lyapunov exponents (Burdet et al., 2006), Shannon's entropy (Lopes & Tenreiro Machado, 2019), approximate entropy (Fonseca, Milho, Passos, Araújo, & Davids, 2012), and sample entropy (Menayo, Encarnación, Gea, & Marcos, 2014), were adopted to study the human performance. Contrarily to traditional methods for variability analysis, such as the standard variation and the coefficient of variation, non-linear methods can provide additional information about the structure of the variability that evolves over time (Couceiro, Clemente, Martins, & Machado, 2014).

Among the many variability analysis methods, the sample entropy is perhaps one of the simplest to compute, while still being one of the most unbiased entropy-related measures (Richman & Moorman, 2000). It is noteworthy that, regardless of the approach, entropy-related metrics can be applied to any other spatio-temporal domain beyond the kinematical analysis, such as in physiological measures (Lake, Richman, Griffin, & Moorman, 2002). However, by trajectory entropy, one implies the employment of this metric, more specifically the sample entropy (*SampEn*), to the trajectory of the athlete and its inherent uncertainty or variability.

The techniques for estimating the sample entropy can be considered as a process represented by a time series and related statistics (Richman & Moorman, 2000). Since the sample entropy can only be applied to a unidimensional time series, the position of player i in the field, previously identified as $x_i[t]$, is decomposed in its dimensions – herein simplified to the xy-plane of the football field, i.e., $x_i[t] = (x_i[t], y_i[t])$. To avoid writing the same equations for both dimensions, let us consider a generic time series $u_i[t]$ to be representative of either $x_i[t]$ or $y_i[t]$. This leads to a sequence of vectors $u_i[1], u_i[2], \ldots, u_i[M-m+1] \in R^{1 \times m}$, each one defined by the array $u_{mi}[k] = \left[u_i[k] u_i[k+1] \cdots u_i[k+m-1] \right]$, $1 \leq k \leq M-m+1$. M, m, and ε are constants, with M being the length of the time series, m the length of sequences to be compared, and ε the tolerance calculated as a percentage of the standard deviation of the data being processed.

A distance between the sequence of vectors $u_{mi}[k]$ can be generally defined as follows:

$$d_{u_i} = \max_{0 \le k \le m-1} \left| u_i[k_1+k] - u_i[k_2+k] \right| \tag{4.4}$$

Let $B_{k_1 i}$ and $A_{k_1 i}$ be, respectively, the number of vectors $u_{mi}[k_2]$ within ε of $u_{mi}[k_1]$ and $u_{m+1i}[k_2]$ within ε of $u_{m+1i}[k_1]$, with $1 \le k \le M-m$, $k_1 \ne k_2$. With this, one can define:

$$\left\{ \begin{array}{l} B_{k_1 i}^m(\varepsilon) = \dfrac{B_{k_1 i}}{M-m+1} \\[3mm] A_{k_1 i}^m(\varepsilon) = \dfrac{A_{k_1 i}}{M-m+1} \end{array} \right. \tag{4.5}$$

and their average as

$$\left\{ \begin{array}{l} B_i^m(\varepsilon) = (M-m+1)^{-1} \displaystyle\sum_{k=1}^{M-m} B_{k\,i}^m(\varepsilon) \\[5mm] A_i^m(\varepsilon) = (M-m+1)^{-1} \displaystyle\sum_{k=1}^{M-m} A_{k\,i}^m(\varepsilon) \end{array} \right. \tag{4.6}$$

Considering a finite length of the time series M, the sample entropy of player i can then be calculated as follows:

$$\text{SampEn}_i(m, \varepsilon) = -\ln\left[\frac{A_i^m(\varepsilon)}{B_i^m(\varepsilon)} \right] \tag{4.7}$$

Libraries and scripts to calculate the sample entropy of a time series are available to the community, as is the case of Martínez–Cagigal's SampEn[1] (Martínez–Cagigal, 2018).

Fractional Dynamics

It may sound like a misconception referring to a dynamics-related metric in a section addressing kinematics. However, it is not. This section has presented a set of computational metrics revolving around the kinematics of the athlete, i.e., metrics that were computed based on the motion of the athlete or its body segments, without considering the forces that cause them to move. This section is no different since the concept of fractional dynamics implies the use of fractional calculus to describe the trajectory of football players, therefore ignoring any forces leading inherent to it.

Only a few numbers of applications based on fractional calculus have been reported so far within sport sciences literature. One of them was the development of a correction metric for golf putting to prevent the inaccurate performance of golfers when facing the golf lip out phenomenon (Couceiro, Dias, Martins, & Luz, 2012). The authors extended a performance metric using the Grünwald-Letnikov approximate discrete equation to integrate a memory of the ball's trajectory. The same authors further applied the concept of fractional calculus in football, be it to improve the accuracy of tracking methods by estimating the position of players based on their trajectory so far (Couceiro, Clemente, & Martins, 2013) and to characterize the predictability and stability levels of players during an official football match (Couceiro, Clemente, Martins, & Machado, 2014).

The previous sections supported the idea that football is a complex dynamic system, wherein the motion of each player is usually chaotic and difficult to predict (Grehaigne, Bouthier, & David, 1997). Under those assumptions and taking into account that the fractional derivative can be considered as a natural extension, or generalization, of the integer (i.e., classical) derivative, it presents itself as an excellent instrument for the description of ecological memory and hereditary properties of processes (i.e., path dependency).

To start with, let us consider the discrete case in which the motion of player i may be defined as follows:

$$x_i[t+1] - x_i[t] = v_i[t+1] \tag{4.8}$$

in such a way that the difference between the position of player i at time $t+1$ and time t, for a period of 1 second, is equal to its current velocity vector $v_i[t+1]$. Hence, $x_i[t+1] - x_i[t]$ corresponds to the first-order integer difference. By adopting the approximate discrete-time Grünwald-Letnikov fractional difference of order $\alpha_i[t]$, generalized to a real number $0 < \alpha_i[t] < 1$, and for a sampling period of 1 second and a truncation order r, the position of player i at time $t+1$ can be written as (Couceiro, Clemente, & Martins, 2013) follows:

$$x_i'[t+1] = x_i[0] + x_i[t] - x_i[t-1] - \sum_{k=1}^{r} \frac{(-1)^k \, \Gamma[\alpha_i[t]+1]}{\Gamma[k+1]\Gamma[\alpha_i[t]-k+1]} x_i[t+1-k] \tag{4.9}$$

with Γ being the gamma function and $x_i'[t+1]$ being the approximated position of player i at time $t+1$. It should be noted that such strategy increases the memory complexity as it requires memorizing the last r positions of each player, i.e.,

$O[rN_\delta]$. Nonetheless, the truncation order r does not need to be too large and will always be inferior to the current time t, i.e., $r \le t$.

As one may observe in Equation (4.12), a problem arises regarding the calculation of the fractional coefficient $\alpha_i[t]$. A player's trajectory can only be correctly defined by adjusting the fractional coefficient $\alpha_i[t]$ along time. In other words, $\alpha_i[t]$ will vary from player to player and over time. Hence, one should find out the best fitting $\alpha_i[t]$ for player i at time t based on its last known positions so far. The value of $\alpha_i[t]$ will be the one that yields a smaller error between the approximated position $x_i'[t+1]$ and the real one $x_i[t+1]$, denoted as $d_i^{\min}$. This reasoning may be formulated by the following minimization problem:

$$s.t\alpha_i[t+1] \in [0,1]. \tag{4.10}$$

The solution of Equation (4.13) can be found with any optimization method, such as golden section search and parabolic interpolation (Brent, 1973; Forsythe, Malcolm, & Moler, 1977). By analysing the effect of $\alpha_i[t]$ in Equation (4.2), one can conclude that the closer to 1 the values of $\alpha_i[t]$ are, the higher predictable player i is. In other words, a value of $\alpha_i[t]=1$ means that Equation (4.12) can accurately predict the next position based on the previous ones, i.e., $x_i'[t+1] = x_i[t+1] \therefore d_i^{\min}(\alpha_i[t]) = 0$. Therefore, for constant and linear trajectories, i.e., without moving at all or with constant speed, the fractional coefficient $\alpha_i[t]$ gets closer to a constant value of 1 – being highly predictable. For a chaotic trajectory, the fractional coefficient variability decreases considerably, presenting values close to $\alpha_i[t]=0.4$ in some situations. This variability is only exceeded by the random trajectories, in which the fractional coefficient in some situations may even get close to $\alpha_i[t]=0$ (Couceiro, Clemente, Martins, & Machado, 2014).

Physiologic Metrics

Many physiologic indicators can help a physiologist to interpret and predict how athletes will react to a certain load. These can be divided into two major categories: (i) invasive methods, and (ii) non-invasive methods. The former can only be assessed with blood parameters, being impractical in a dynamic environment at the current state of the technology. As this book revolves around the topic of pattern recognition in sports during training and competition, the focus will be placed on the latter. In non-invasive physiological methods, one can assess many variables that can help to better understand how the athlete is reacting to the loads without blood parameters and, at the same time, maintaining the ecological circumstances of performance in obtaining the data by employing technologies that do not perturb the athlete. This section includes the description of basic physiological features, such as **heart rate** and muscle activity (**electromyography**). These are examples of physiological data generated by the human body from which it is possible to assess a person's stress, which may be perceived not always consciously nor through non-physiological data (Jerritta, Murugappan, Nagarajan, & Wan, 2011). All this is possible due to the ability to draw more representative features from these signals, such as the **mean heart rate variability, muscle load**, and other related metrics obtained through signal processing, such as **electromyography root mean square** and **electromyography Fourier transform**.

Heart Rate

Heart rate (HR) reflects the number of systoles that occurs per minute, caused by the activity of the parasympathetic and sympathetic nervous system in the sinus node. These systems work in search of balance, since the sympathetic system is responsible for the body's responses to certain impulses, making the heart rhythm to meet the necessary requirements. The parasympathetic system, however, is responsible for the heart response when at rest (HR between 60 and 100 beats per minute) and also the one that assumes the relaxation function by slowing the HR when facing an increased activity.

The resting heart rhythm (HR_{rest}) represents the basal heart rhythm and should, therefore, be measured after awakening and preferably in an isolated space where the person suffers as little disturbance as possible. In athletes, this tends to decrease with aerobic training, so it is of high importance to know this metric for each athlete in order to be able to evaluate his/her performance or to make the screening of any health problem. The maximum heart rhythm (HR_{max}) is reached when the athlete is under a high physical load, forcing the body to request as much oxygen as possible, causing the number of systoles to reach a maximum. Through these two concepts, it is possible to obtain the heart rate reserve (HR_R) for player i as follows:

$$HR_{Ri} = HR_{maxi} - HR_{resti} \qquad (4.11)$$

Given the current heart rate values of a player i, $HR_i[t]$, which can be extracted with state-of-the-art heart rate monitors (see Chapter 3), and considering that HR_{maxi} and HR_{resti} are known constant values, the heart rate values can be normalized for each time step t by applying the following equation:

$$HR_{normi}[t] = \frac{HR_i[t] - HR_{resti}}{HR_{maxi} - HR_{resti}} \qquad (4.12)$$

Besides heart rate, the heart rate variability (HRV) is often adopted to monitor training loads. The analysis of HVR can be made by computing a time series of RR intervals, i.e., the intervals between successive heartbeats, or R waves. If updated at every timestamp t for each player i, the time series RR can be expressed as a time-varying variable $RR_i[t]$. This can, once again, be tracked with wearable technologies, such as heart rate monitor chest bands. With $RR_i[t]$ as an available feature, one can calculate multiple additional physiological metrics. These metrics, however, since they rely on average measurements, shall only be updated at every integer number of steps t (e.g., every second). The mean heart rate variability ($mHRV_i[t]$) is the most common metric, being calculated as the simple moving average of $RR_i[t]$:

$$mHRV_i[t] = \frac{1}{t} \sum_{k=1,k\in N}^{t} RR_i[k] \tag{4.13}$$

The standard deviation of all NN intervals (normal RR intervals), known as $SDNN_i[t]$, indicates the global HRV and can be calculated as follows:

$$SDNN_i[t] = \sqrt{\frac{\sum_{k=1,k\in N}^{t} \left(RR_i[k] - mHRV_i[k]\right)^2}{t-1}} \tag{4.14}$$

The root mean square of the successive differences in RR intervals ($RMSSD_i[t]$) allows estimating variations in heart rate in short-term RR recordings, being calculated as follows:

$$RMSSD_i[t] = \sqrt{\frac{1}{t} \sum_{k=1}^{t-1} \left(RR_i[k+1] - RR_i[k]\right)^2} \tag{4.15}$$

Electromyography

Any movement performed by the human body implies a certain muscular effort, however small it may be. Whether it is a contraction, concentric, eccentric, or isometric, the muscle generates electrical potentials that are studied through electromyography (EMG) (Konrad, 2005). Measuring on the surface of the skin, known as surface electromyography (sEMG), has particular interest for rehabilitation, sports, and even ergonomics (Vigotsky, Halperin, Lehman, Trajano, & Vieira, 2018).

The acquisition of the EMG signal can be made through conductor electrodes or conductive fabric that must be applied to the groups of muscles to be measured. Within the context of football, it is necessary to take into account the comfort of the athlete on choosing the most appropriate technology and, above all, to focus on the muscles that might be more participative in the task: the lower limbs. A few solutions have been made available in the market for this purpose, as is the case of *Myontec MBody 3*, which allows collecting multiple channels of muscle activity in the legs. The muscle activity of a given player i can be quantified by the amplitude value of the signal, $A_i^{ch}[t]$, of a given channel ch out of a total number of channels ch_{tot}.

Yet, even if multiple channels might be available, most of the time, additional features still need to be computed out of EMG data, employing pre-processing routines, including filtering, rectification, and smoothing (Merletti & Di Torino, 1999). Filtering is intended to remove unwanted noise from the original signal. In some cases, when the acquisition device returns clean signals, this process is not necessary. However, when there is a need to filter, a band-pass filter is usually applied, removing both low and high frequencies. The removal of the low frequencies eliminates the baseline deviation which is usually associated with slight movements and even breathing, with typical frequency values of 5–20 Hz. The high-frequency cut-off prevents the occurrence of signal aliasing, with typical values between 200 Hz and 1 kHz. With the rectification, a reorganization of the signal is made to calculate standard amplitude parameters, such as average, peak values, and area. Basically, all negative amplitudes are converted to positive amplitudes. It should be noted that, unlike filtering, this procedure does not affect signal noise, so smoothing may be necessary. Through smoothing, it is possible to create a linear envelope of the signal, leaving only a centred part of it. Usually, a Butterworth filter is used, which is a low-pass filter, being considered one of the best digital filters to decrease the relationship between signal and noise (Mello, Oliveira, & Nadal, 2007).

Muscle Load

One of the features that can be computed directly through the acquisition of EMG signal is the muscle load of player i at time $ML_i[t]$. This feature translates the sum of all the data coming from the different monitored muscle groups at each instant:

$$ML_i[t] = \sum_{ch=1}^{ch_{tot}} A_i^{ch}[t] \qquad (4.16)$$

The muscle balance quantifies the distribution of the muscle activity between the left $B_i^L[t]$ and right $B_i^R[t]$ sides of the body. If we consider that the first half of the EMG channels represent the left leg and the other half the right leg, the balance-related metrics can be calculated as follows:

$$B_i^L[t] = \frac{\sum_{ch=1}^{ch_{tot}/2} A_i^{ch}[t]}{\sum_{ch=1}^{ch_{tot}} A_i^{ch}[t]}$$

$$B_i^R[t] = \frac{\sum_{\frac{ch_{tot}}{2}+1}^{ch_{tot}} A_i^{ch}[t]}{\sum_{ch=1}^{ch_{tot}} A_i^{ch}[t]} \qquad (4.17)$$

Still in the same domain, it is possible to retrieve the effort of a given muscle tracked by a given channel ch when compared to the global effort, which provides insights about the muscle distribution as follows:

$$D_i^{ch}[t] = \frac{A_i^{ch}[t]}{\sum_{ch=1}^{ch_{tot}} A_i^{ch}[t]} \tag{4.18}$$

Electromyography Root Mean Square

The root mean square of an EMG signal from a given channel, $EMG_{RMSi}^{ch}[t]$, has been often adopted to quantify the electric signal because it reflects the physiological activity in the motor unit during contraction (Fukuda et al., 2010). Put it differently, the $EMG_{RMSi}^{ch}[t]$ shows the variations in the strength of athlete i over time t (Chai & Draxler, 2014), which can be mathematically represented as follows:

$$EMG_{RMSi}^{ch}[t] = \sqrt{\frac{1}{t}\sum_{k=1}^{t} A_i^{ch}[k]^2} \tag{4.19}$$

While there is a relationship between the root mean square of an EMG signal and the force employed by the athlete, such relationship tends to be more linear for small muscles (Basmajian, 1962). Larger muscles that need better motor recruitment lead to non-linear relationships between force and EMG signal because the amplitude variations of the muscle electric signal do not correspond to the force variations. Therefore, it is necessary to go beyond the time analysis of EMG signals, stepping into the frequency domain, where the signal energy is distributed over a range of frequencies, being, for instance, an added value for predicting muscle fatigue.

Electromyography Fourier Transform

The most popular method for converting a signal from a time domain to a frequency domain is the Fourier transform. It allows decomposing a function into the sum of a, potentially infinite, number of sine wave frequency components. As such, when performing the Fourier transform of a signal, two outputs are provided: the magnitude and the power spectrum (Proakis & Manolakis, 1996). When the Fourier transform is applied to the EMG signal A_i^{ch}, this one goes from the set of real numbers to the set of complex numbers $R \to C$, so the signal is written by the sum of its real number a and its imaginary number jb.

Let n_t be the number of samples of an EMG signal $A_i^{ch}[t]$ for player i and channel ch; its FFT is a length n_t vector $EMG_{FFTi}^{ch}[f]$ for a given frequency f, as is shown in the following equation:

$$EMG_{FFTi}^{ch}[f] = \sum_{t=0}^{n_t-1} A_i^{ch}[t] e^{-j2\pi f \frac{t}{n_t}}$$

(4.20)

According to the literature, the sampling frequency of an EMG signal is typically 1 kHz, which allows capturing the entire frequency range of the signal. The 'usable' part of the signal's energy has a frequency between 0 Hz and 500 Hz and the dominant energy part falls on a frequency between 50 Hz and 150 Hz (De Luca, 2002). This implies that while $EMG_{FFTi}^{ch}[f]$ needs to be calculated for each time t, as it depends on $A_i^{ch}[t]$, it also means that it shall be computed for a given frequency or range of frequencies f. This may lead to more than one series for each time t and, as a consequence, to multiple sequence data features.

Group Metrics

As stated on multiple occasions before, football is a collective dynamic system that encompasses interactions between players. Those interactions can be, to some extent, measured by employing and analysing the positional data (Clemente, Sequeiros, Correia, Silva, & Martins, 2018), though more is needed to understand how the team organizes itself to achieve the aim of scoring (Grehaigne et al., 1997). Measuring the individual positional data, however, makes it possible to compute other variables able to provide valuable information about the behaviour of the team (Duarte, Araújo, Correia, & Davids, 2012). This may allow coaches to make more efficient strategic decisions, either before or during matches (Clemente et al., 2018).

The perception of how collective teams behave, by identifying strengths and weaknesses, is of the utmost importance for coaches. The understanding of how to organize all the players is, in fact, a challenge (Couceiro, Clemente, Dias et al., 2014). Analysing patterns among players, similarly to the analysis of individual behaviour, can give coaches and sports analysts metrics that can represent how all players perform during matches. A group measurement system, however, be it from collective sports, swarm intelligence, multi-robot systems, or any other domain, inherently offers a high analysis complexity, which usually grows as the number of competitive agents grows (Navarro & Matía, 2009; Tsai, 2002). For instance, in a football match, we may be facing a group system comprising 11 cooperative agents competing against other 11 cooperative agents. How the coordination of these athletes emerges is a basic problem in the performance analysis of team sports (Araújo & Davids, 2016). Individuals from the same team must play together as a team, which may call upon maintaining certain relative positions among them and the opposing team. Metrics relying on the position of players in the field fall in the tactical analysis domain (Clemente, Couceiro, Martins, Mendes, & Figueiredo, 2013).

Nonetheless, group systems, including team sports, are characterized by more than agents' position, often offering rich dynamic interactions able to shape the outcome (e.g., the end result of the match). In team sports, interactions between players of the same team are fostered with the intent to undermine the objectives of the opposing team, while fulfilling their own objectives (Cliff et al., 2013). This leads to complex spatio-temporal interactions, which may seem intractable to understand and quantify. While the position of players in the field does play a role in such interactions, it is necessary to consider the more directed nature of such correlations, where the overall dynamics of the team is affected by the dynamics of each individual. Due to the nature of the players' interactive behaviours (involving teammates and opponents), football, more than other team sports, has been characterized as involving great variability and unpredictability of actions, leading researchers to investigate the **networks** of interactions that emerge among football players within teams (Gama et al., 2014; Vilar et al., 2014). Next sections further explore tactical variables obtained from spatial-temporal (positional) and **networks** metrics.

Spatial-Temporal Metrics

Online spatial-temporal metrics may provide relevant information about how teams, as a collective system, behave over time throughout the match (Clemente et al., 2013). In fact, such metrics can be used as an important tool to improve the coaching opportunities to make changes on the team's strategy, allowing detecting and acting upon its weaknesses during the match. For this, the **weighted centroid**, **weighted stretch index**, and **surface area** are hereby described.

Weighted Centroid

In football and all other team sports, the centroid is often calculated through the geometric mean position of all players of a given team. As before, the position of player i in the field is decomposed in its dimensions as $x_i[t] = (x_i[t], y_i[t])$. Then, the centroid $\left(x'[t], y'[t]\right)$ can be calculated based on the geometric position of all N players $(x_i[t], y_i[t])$ for each team. According to Frencken and Lemmink (2008), the centroid provides three relevant measurements: (i) the x-distance, representing forward-backward displacement (i.e., length of the field); (ii) the y-distance, representing lateral displacement (i.e., width of the field); and (iii) the radial distance, comprising both forward-backward and lateral displacements. These are obtained based on the centroid position relative to the origin O, i.e., $(0,0)$, defined at the centre of the field, as follows:

$$
\begin{bmatrix} x'[t] \\ y'[t] \end{bmatrix} = \frac{1}{\sum_{i=1}^{N} w_i[t]} \begin{bmatrix} \sum_{i=1}^{N} w_i[t] x_i[t] \\ \sum_{i=1}^{N} w_i[t] y_i[t] \end{bmatrix}
\tag{4.21}
$$

wherein the position of the ith player is defined as $(x_i[t],\ y_i[t])$ and $w_i[t]$ is the weighting factor of such player. Many studies do not consider the positions of the goalkeeper and the ball (Bourbousson, Sève, & McGarry, 2010; Frencken, Lemmink, Delleman, & Visscher, 2011). Nevertheless, both should be considered for different reasons: the goalkeeper due to his/her preponderance in the defensive phase, and the ball since the player's influence shall decrease with the distance to it. In other words, the relevance of the ith player to the team's centroid, i.e., $w_i[t][t]$, is based on the Euclidean distance from the ith player to the ball as follows:

$$
w_i[t] = 1 - \frac{\sqrt{\left(x_i[t] - x_b[t]\right)^2 + \left(y_i[t] - y_b[t]\right)^2}}{d_{\max}[t]}
\tag{4.22}
$$

where $(x_b[t],\ y_b[t])$ corresponds to the position of the ball and $d_{\max}[t]$ is the Euclidean distance of the farthest player to the ball at each time t (Figure 4.1).

Weighted Stretch Index

The stretch index measures the space expansion or contraction of the team on the longitudinal and lateral directions (Bourbousson, Sève, et al., 2010).

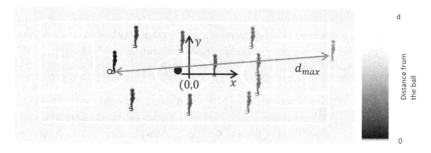

FIGURE 4.1 Spatial referential of the field (Clemente et al., 2013).

Similarly to the team's centroid, the weighted team's stretch index may be calculated as follows:

$$s_{ind}[t] = \frac{\sum_{i=1}^{N} w_i[t] d_i[t]}{\sum_{i=1}^{N} w_i[t]} \qquad (4.23)$$

where $d_i[t]$ is the Euclidean distance between player i and the team's centroid, which is expressed as follows:

$$d_i[t] = \sqrt{\left(x_i[t] - x'[t]\right)^2 + \left(y_i[t] - y'[t]\right)^2} \qquad (4.24)$$

Put it differently, the stretch index can be obtained by computing the mean of the distances between each player and the centroid of the team. Hence, this metric represents the mean deviation of each player on a team from its centroid.

Effective Surface Area

Computing an effective surface area, also known as team coverage area, and as opposed to the majority of the works presented in the literature (e.g., Moura, Martins, Anido, De Barros, & Cunha, 2012), is more complex than the previous tactical metrics. To create a polygon on the planar dimension, i.e., a triangle, at least three points are necessary. Therefore, three players need to be considered to build triangles as the combinations of N players (in which, as stated earlier, N is the total number of players within a team). On the football case, a maximum of 11 players for each team may be in the field at the same time. Consequently, the combination of three out of eleven players results in a total of 165 triangles that may be cumulatively formed (Algorithm 4.1).

Algorithm 4.1.   Calculate the surface area of the team.

$l = 0$ // counter of the combinations of N players taken three at a time

For $i = 1 : N - 2$

    For $j = i + 1 : N - 1$

        For $k = j + 1 : N$

            $l = l + 1$

            $\Delta_l = \begin{bmatrix} x_i & x_j & x_k \\ y_i & y_j & y_k \end{bmatrix}^T$ // each triangle is defined by the position

            of three different players

$P = \Delta_1$ // initialize the polygon as the first triangle defined by players 1, 2, and 3

For $i = 2 : l$

$\quad \left| \begin{array}{l} P = P \cup \Delta_i, \text{ where } P = \left(p_1, \ldots, p_\alpha \right) \wedge \alpha \leq N \text{ // build the polygon by} \\ \text{accumulatively uniting itself to the remaining triangles} \end{array} \right.$

$A_{Pol} = \dfrac{1}{2} \displaystyle\sum_{i=1}^{\alpha-1} \left(p_{1,i} p_{2,i+1} - p_{1,i+1} p_{2,i} \right)$, with $\alpha \leq N$ // calculate the area of the polygon

---

The concept of effective play area comes from Gréhaigne (1993), defining it as the instant peripheral position of players. That is to say that the surface area should contemplate the effective available space a team can play. Therefore, the effective area of a team should be modelled as the real area that a team covers without intercepting the effective area of the opposing team. This requires a more thorough geometrical analysis of the tactical football strategy to further understand how teams behave over time.

Triangles formed between players are known to be the geometric figures leading to the most successful play along the field (Lucchesi, 2001). The ability of the team to 'draw up' such triangles on the field allows developing a good offensive (Clemente et al., 2013). Also, defensive triangles are always being formed in an attempt to create a 'defensive shadow', i.e., space through which the opponent cannot pass or dibble due to the triangular-shaped positioning of players (Dooley & Titz, 2010). With this in mind, Algorithm 4.2 calculates all

---

Algorithm 4.2. Calculate the surface area of team δ with non-overlapping triangles.

$l^\delta = 0$ // counter of the combinations of N players of team δ taken three at a time

For $i = 1 : N^\delta - 2$

$\quad \left| \begin{array}{l} \text{For } j = i+1 : N^\delta - 1 \\[4pt] \quad \left| \begin{array}{l} \text{For } k = j+1 : N^\delta \\[4pt] \quad \left| \begin{array}{l} l^\delta = l^\delta + 1 \\[6pt] \Delta_l^\delta = \begin{bmatrix} x_i & x_j & x_k \\ y_i & y_j & y_k \end{bmatrix}^T \quad \text{// each triangle is defined by the position} \\[6pt] \text{of three different players} \\[6pt] \rho_l = \displaystyle\sum_{i=1}^{3} \left(x_i - x_j, \, y_i - y_j \right) \|, \text{ with } i \neq j \wedge i < j \end{array} \right. \end{array} \right. \end{array} \right.$

$$\vec{s} = sort_{ascending}\left(\vec{p}\right) \in R^{1 \times \beta}, \text{ where } \vec{p} = \left(\rho_1, \ldots, \rho_\alpha\right) \wedge \beta = \binom{N^\delta}{3}$$

$P^\delta = \Delta_{s_1}^\delta$ // initialize the polygon as the triangle with the smallest perimeter

$\Delta_1^\delta = \Delta_{s_1}^\delta$ // initialize the non-overlapping triangles of team δ

$\tau^\delta = 1$ // counter of the non-overlapping triangles of team δ

For $i = 2 : I^\delta$

$\Gamma = P^\delta \cap \Delta_i^\delta$, where $\Gamma = \left(\gamma_1, \ldots, \gamma_\alpha\right) \wedge \alpha \leq N^\delta$ // analyse intersections between triangles

$$A_{Pol} = \frac{1}{2} \sum_{i=1}^{\alpha-1} \left(\gamma_{1,i}\gamma_{2,i+1} - \gamma_{1,i+1}\gamma_{2,i}\right) \text{ with } \alpha \leq N^\delta \text{ // calculate the area of the}$$

intersection

If $A_{Pol} = 0$ // condition is verified when there is no intersection between triangles

$\tau^\delta = \tau^\delta + 1$

$P^\delta = P^\delta \cup \Delta_i^\delta$ // build the polygon by accumulatively uniting the non-overlapping triangles

$\Delta_{\tau^\delta}^\delta = \Delta_i^\delta$ // non-overlapping τ^δ triangle of team δ

the non-overlapping triangles formed by players of the same team, generating, at first, the triangles with smaller perimeters.

Trapattoni (2000) claims that, when players are pressed and cannot turn around and dribble, the ball must travel along with triangles until a solution is found, i.e., the offensive triangles are annulled by the defensive triangles. Put it differently, as the number of formed triangles within a team increases, the less effective space is left for the opposing team. Hence, after generating all triangles of each team, Algorithm 4.3 computes the triangles of each team that do not suffer from the intersection of the opposing team, subsequently allowing to calculate the area of each team without an interception.

In Algorithm 4.3, both teams are simultaneously considered, in which δ and ζ are the team superscript, such that $\delta = \{1,2\}$ and $\zeta = \{1,2\}$, with $\delta \neq \zeta$. However, in the presence of interceptions between opposing triangles, and based on the supposition that effective defensive triangles can overlap the offensive triangles (Trapattoni, 2000), the effective area to be considered is one of the defensive triangles (Figure 4.2a), thus reducing the effective area of the offensive team.

Algorithm 4.3. Effective Area – Triangles of team δ that do not intersect the surface area of the opposing team ζ.

$\varepsilon^\delta = 0$ // counter of the effective triangles of team δ

$A^\delta = 0$ // effective area of team δ

$E^\delta = [\ ]$ // polygon of the effective area of team δ is initialized as an empty array

For $i = 1 : \tau^\delta$

> $\Gamma = \Delta_i^\delta \cap P^\zeta$, where $\Gamma = (\gamma_1, \ldots, \gamma_\alpha) \wedge \alpha \leq 6$ // analyse intersections between triangles
>
> $A_{Pol} = \dfrac{1}{2} \displaystyle\sum_{i=1}^{\alpha-1} \left(\gamma_{1,i}\gamma_{2,i+1} - \gamma_{1,i+1}\gamma_{2,i} \right)$ with $\alpha \leq 6$ // calculate the area of the intersection
>
> If $A_{Pol} = 0$ // condition is verified when there is no intersection between the triangle from team δ and the surface area of team ζ
>
> > $A_{Pol} = \dfrac{1}{2} \displaystyle\sum_{i=1}^{3} \left(x_i y_{i+1} - x_{i+1} y_i \right)$ // calculate the area of the triangle
> >
> > $A^\delta = A^\delta + A_{Pol}$ // cumulative effective area of team δ
> >
> > $\varepsilon^\delta = \varepsilon^\delta + 1$ // counter of the effective triangles of team δ
> >
> > $E^\delta = E^\delta \cup \Delta_i^\delta$ // build the polygon of the effective area of team δ by accumulatively uniting its effective triangles

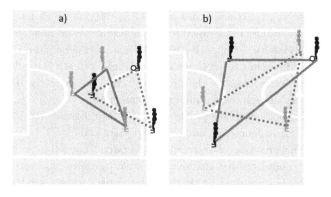

FIGURE 4.2 Example of triangles interception (Clemente et al., 2013).

According to Dooley and Titz (2010), effective defensive triangles in football can only be established if defensive players are able to ensure a maximum distance of 12 m between them. Generalizing this rationale, an offensive triangle will overlap a defensive triangle with a perimeter above 36 m since there are no guarantees that the defensive players will be able to intercept the ball (Figure 4.2b). It is noteworthy that this rationale takes into account the specific football dynamics and that effective defensive formations from other team sports will inevitably lead to changes in the algorithm. However, to keep it as generalized as possible, the maximum perimeter of the triangle is defined by ρ_ε which, for this particular case, is set to $\rho_\varepsilon = 36$. With this in mind, Algorithm 4.4 considers that all triangles of the defensive team with perimeter inferior to 36 m overlap the interceptive offensive triangles (Algorithm 4.4).

Algorithm 4.4. Effective Area – Defensive triangles of team δ that intersect the surface area of the opposing team ζ.

If $ball_{possession}(\zeta) = 1$ // condition is verified when team ζ has the possession of the ball

For $i = 1 : \tau^\delta$

$\Gamma = \Delta_i^\delta \cap P^\zeta$, where $\Gamma = (\gamma_1, ..., \gamma_\alpha) \wedge \alpha \leq 6$ // analyse intersections between triangles

$$A_{Pol} = \frac{1}{2} \sum_{i=1}^{\alpha-1} (\gamma_{1,i}\gamma_{2,i+1} - \gamma_{1,i+1}\gamma_{2,i}) \text{ with } \alpha \leq 6 \text{ // calculate the area of the}$$ intersection

$$\rho_{Pol} = \sum_{i=1}^{3} (x_i - x_j, \ y_i - y_j), \text{ with } i \neq j \wedge i < j$$

If $A_{Pol} > 0 \wedge \rho_{Pol} \leq \rho_\varepsilon$ // condition is verified when there is an intersection between the defensive triangle from team δ and the surface area of team ζ and the perimeter of the defensive triangle is smaller than ρ_ε

$$A_{Pol} = \frac{1}{2} \sum_{i=1}^{3} (x_i y_{i+1} - x_{i+1} y_i) \text{ // calculate the area of the triangle}$$

$A^\delta = A^\delta + A_{Pol}$ // cumulative effective area of team δ

$\varepsilon^\delta = \varepsilon^\delta + 1$ // counter of the effective triangles of team δ

$P^\delta = P^\delta \cup \Delta_i^\delta$ // build the polygon of the effective area of team δ by accumulatively uniting its effective triangles

At last, Algorithm 4.5 takes into account all offensive triangles that are not intercepted by the defensive triangles with perimeter inferior to $\rho_\varepsilon = 36$ m, leading to the effective areas of both teams at every instant.

Algorithm 4.5. Effective Area – Offensive triangles of team δ that are not intersected by the defensive triangles of the opposing team ζ.

If $ball_{possession}(\delta) = 1$ // condition is verified when team δ has the possession of the ball

For $i = 1 : \tau^\delta$

$$\Gamma = \Delta_i^\delta \cap \left(P^\delta \bigcup P^\zeta \right), \text{ where } \Gamma = (\gamma_\alpha \ldots, \gamma_\alpha) \wedge \alpha \leq 6 \text{ // analyse}$$

intersections between offensive triangles and the effective area of both teams

$$A_{Pol} = \frac{1}{2} \sum_{i=1}^{\alpha-1} \left(\gamma_{1,i}\gamma_{2,i+1} - \gamma_{1,i+1}\gamma_{2,i} \right) \text{ with } \alpha \leq 6 \text{ // calculate the area of the}$$

intersection

If $A_{Pol} = 0$ // condition is verified when there is an intersection between the defensive triangle from team δ and the surface area of team ζ and the perimeter of the defensive triangle is smaller than ρ_ε

$$A_{Pol} = \frac{1}{2} \sum_{i=1}^{3} \left(x_i y_{i+1} - x_{i+1} y_i \right) \text{ // calculate the area of the triangle}$$

$$A^\delta = A^\delta + A_{Pol} \text{ // cumulative effective area of team } \delta$$

$$\varepsilon^\delta = \varepsilon^\delta + 1 \text{ // counter of the effective triangles of team } \delta$$

$$P^\delta = P^\delta \cup \Delta_i^\delta \text{ // build the polygon of the effective area of team } \delta \text{ by}$$
accumulatively uniting its effective triangles

The effective surface area of the polygon $P^\delta[t]$ formed by team δ is computed at each time t, $A^\delta[t]$, with the same being done for team ζ. This is illustrated in Figure 4.3, in which the offensive formation from team δ is being intercepted by a set of efficient defensive triangles. This allows analysing if a team, in the defensive phase, acts as a defensive 'block', i.e., the union ($\cup$) of the defensive triangles forms a defensive polygon that constrains the opponents to lose the ball. It also allows analysing if the midfielders' triangles are large enough to allow offensive triangle moving forward without effective opposition. Additionally, to the team's effective area, the number of effective triangles of each team may characterize the efficiency of the team's tactical organization.

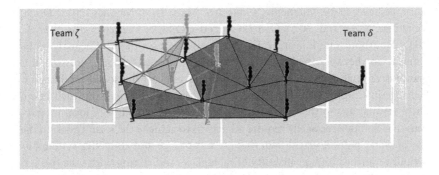

FIGURE 4.3 Example of effective area with defensive and offensive effective triangles.

Put together, the effective area and the number of triangles can give different and complementary information, since a team with the same number of effective triangles may have a different effective area in different situations.

Just like all other computational metrics presented in this chapter, the computation of the effective area needs to be undertaken in real time (while the football match is running), which, considering its complexity, calls upon high-performing computers and an efficient selection of certain subroutines. Before computing the team's effective area, one needs to compute the surface area with non-overlapping triangles (Algorithm 4.2). To form a triangle between the players from team δ, a three combination of the N^δ players may be considered as a subset of three distinct players of N^δ. The time complexity to compute the team's surface area is further increased as one also needs to sort the perimeters of all triangles (cf., Algorithm 4.2). For a list of a computationally efficient sorting algorithm, refer to Bhalchandra, Deshmukh, Lokhande, and Phulari (2009).

The team's effective area is then divided into three algorithms. Algorithms 4.3 and 4.4 linearly depend on the number of non-overlapping triangles from team δ, i.e., τ^δ. However, Algorithm 4.5 depends on the number of non-overlapping triangles from the opposing team, i.e., τ^ζ. Moreover, the computation from the effective area from both teams depends on one another. At last, integrating all metrics, the computing requirements, for both teams, can be mathematically described as follows:

$$O\left(3\binom{N^\delta}{3} + 3\binom{N^\zeta}{3} + 3\left(\tau^\delta + \tau^\zeta\right) + 2\left(N^\delta + N^\zeta\right)\right) \qquad (4.25)$$

Networks Metrics

The sports literature offers a wide range of approaches exploring graph theory, in which graphs are used to represent networks (Bourbousson, Poizat,

Saury, & Seve, 2010; Clemente, Couceiro, Martins, & Mendes, 2015; Duch, Waitzman, & Amaral, 2010; Gama, Couceiro, Dias, & Vaz, 2015; Passos et al., 2011). Bourbousson, Poizat et al. (2010) used graph theory to analyse the connectivity between basketball players in each unit of attack, crossing this quantitative analysis with a qualitative one to explain the social interactions. Their main finding was the rise of a specific network regarding each team. These results suggest that a network's coordination was built on local interactions that do not necessarily require all players to achieve the team's goal. In the case of water polo, it was shown that the most successful collective system behaviour requires a high probability of each player interacting with other players in a team (Passos et al., 2011). In football, researchers proposed to analyse the attacking plays that result in shots and identify the main players that contribute to the process of building the attack (Duch et al., 2010). Using a centrality approach, they found the player with the most influence on each analysed team. Such an approach was compared with an observational analysis of experts and showed strong correspondence. Clemente et al. (2015) proposed a set of computational metrics computed on top of networks of offensive football plays. The authors followed a more macroscopic approach than the previous works, dealing with density, heterogeneity, and centralization network metrics, with the intent to identify how players connect with each other during offensive moments. Similarly, Gama et al. (2015) also considered networks formed by offensive plays, which included passes, crosses into the penalty box and ball receptions. However, in Gama et al. (2015), the focus was placed in exploring the concept of small-world networks, focusing on the scaled connectivity between players, the clustering coefficient, and the global rank, suggesting that players' interactive behaviours within a football match support the existence of a scale-free network. A dynamic and multilevel approach, called hypernetworks, was taken by Ramos and colleagues (Ramos, Lopes, & Araújo, 2020; Ramos, Lopes, Marques, & Araújo, 2017; Ribeiro et al., 2019). Hypernetworks simultaneously access cooperative and competitive interactions between teammates and opponents across space and time during a match. Moreover, hypernetworks are not limited to dyadic relations – how sets of players interact with sets of players.

Be it biological, sociological, or any other network for that matter, they all share specific topological properties. From the aforementioned works and many other available in the literature, several useful network concepts from graph theory have been adopted to identify and describe such properties. Network-related computational metrics start with the basic principle of creating a weighted adjacency matrix $A[t] = \left[a_{ij}[t] \right] \in R^{N \times N}$, with N being the number of players of a given team and a_{ij} representing the interaction level established from player i to player j in time t. How such interaction is defined is the key to successfully employ network analysis in team sports.

The vast majority of the works available in the network analysis sports literature associate interactions with passes made from one player to another

(Brandt & Brefeld, 2015). In this context, the interaction $a_{ij}[t]$ can be defined as follows:

$$a_{ij}[t] = \sum_{k=0}^{t} p_{ij}[k]$$ (4.26)

with p_{ij} being defined as 1 whenever a successful pass from player i to player j occurs, and zero otherwise. The diagonal elements (i.e., $i = j$) are set equal to 1 to identify player i as the one performing the pass, which, cumulatively, would also provide a general overview of how many passes in total were carried out by that particular player to all teammates. By adopting a directional approach as this, wherein the link established between players i and j (pass performed by player i to player j) is independent of the link established between j and i (pass performed by player j to player i), directed graphs, or digraphs, are expected to occur (van Den Brink & Borm, 2002). Nonetheless, given the rather more complex analysis inherent to digraphs, many sport scientists separately analyse two undirected graphs: one for each direction of the interaction. Put it differently, if passes are how interactions between players are established, then two networks would be established: one for performed passes, and another for received passes (Gama et al., 2015). This also means two separated adjacency matrices and related variables. For the sake of simplicity, and without loss of generality, let us consider examples of a single graph (or adjacency matrix).

Similarly, other works put a more macroscopic meaning to interactions within the network, where the entries $a_{ij}[t]$ represent the individual participation in the cumulative number of offensive plays until time t (i.e., the network is developed considering the number of consecutive passes until the ball is lost) (Clemente, Couceiro, Martins, & Mendes, 2014). For this particular situation, $a_{ij}[t]$ is set equal to $a_{ji}[t]$, leading to the more traditional undirected graph, focus on the players who contributed to a given offensive play. In this situation, the diagonal elements (i.e., $i = j$) are set equal to 1 to identify the player i as one of the players who participated in the offensive play, which, cumulatively, would also provide a general overview of the contribution given to the team.

From this point, regardless of how interactions between players are quantified, several optimizations can be considered. For instance, the $a_{ij}[t]$ interaction can be normalized, leading to a relative weighted adjacency matrix defined as follows:

$$a_{ij}[t] = \begin{cases} \dfrac{\sum_{k=0}^{t} p_{ij}[k]}{\max_{k,\,l,\,k \neq l} p_{kl}[t]}, & i \neq j \\[2em] \sum_{k=0}^{t} p_{ii}[k], & i = j \end{cases}$$ (4.27)

where $0 \le a_{ij}[t] \le 1$ for $i \ne j$, with $i, j = 1, \ldots, N$. For instance, for interactions defined as passes performed, the denominator $\max_{k, l, k \ne l} p_{kl}[t]$ would correspond to the maximum number of passes performed by a given player, while for offensive actions, it would correspond to the maximum number of offensive plays a given player participated in.

An example of a network based on offensive plays of a given team is illustrated in Figure 4.4 (Clemente et al., 2015). It is noteworthy that 14 players ($N = 14$) have been considered as it encompasses 11 players in the field plus 3 substitutes. Many libraries and scripts to plot these networks have been made available to the scientific community over the past decade. The network illustrated in Figure 4.4 was generated using the wpPlot MATLAB script developed by Wu (2020).[2] For this situation, wpPlot has been further extended based on the following features: (i) the vertex i (i.e., player) size is proportional to the offensive plays player i participates in; (ii) the edge $a_{ij}[t] = a_{ji}[t]$, $i \ne j$, thickness, and colour are directly related to the number of offensive plays in which players i and j cooperate in.

From Figure 4.4, one can visually observe that player 3 (central defender) seems to be key to the offensive plays fulfilled by the team, with the strongest collaborations (thickest edges) being with players 4 (central defender) and 12 (right defender). As expected, by mere observation, it is not possible to quantify how much the player stands out from the remaining team or anything else for that matter. A set of computational metrics needs to be adopted, and the network theory or, more generally, the graph theory is one of the prime objects of study in discrete mathematics. More than being just a visual representation, these metrics may clarify the individual contribution of each player in a given context. Likewise, by using network methodology, it may be possible to identify the players who interact the most with their neighbouring teammates

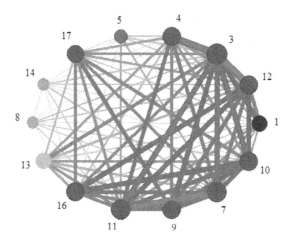

FIGURE 4.4 Network representation of passes between players for a single match comprising 14 football players of a team.

and the ones who contribute the most to successful and unsuccessful collective actions (Clemente et al., 2014; Gama et al., 2014).

It is noteworthy that the subsequent metrics were contextualized considering the network interactions as passes performed. However, as previously addressed, bear in mind that network interactions are abstract links, or edges, connecting vertices (players), which can represent any other quantifiable relationship between them.

Scaled Connectivity

The first analysis and one of the most widely used in the literature for distinguishing a vertex of a network from another is the connectivity, which is also known as degree (Horvath, 2011). Within the football context, the connectivity $c_i[t]$ equals the sum of connection weights between player i and the other players at time t as follows:

$$c_i[t] = \sum_{j=1c, j\neq i}^{N} a_{ij}[t] \tag{4.28}$$

The most cooperative player, or players, can be found by computing the indices of the maximum connectivity:

$$c_{max}[t] = \max_i c_i[t] \tag{4.29}$$

One can then define a relative connectivity, known as scaled connectivity, of player i as follows:

$$sc_i[t] = \frac{c_i[t]}{c_{max}[t]} \tag{4.30}$$

such that $sc = [sc_i] \in R^{1\times N}$ is the vector of the relative connectivity of players. The scaled connectivity represents a measure of the level of cooperation of a given player in which high values of sc_i (i.e., as sc_i tends to 1) indicate that the ith player collaborates with most of the teammates (Clemente et al., 2014).

Clustering Coefficient

The clustering coefficient of player i offers a measure of the degree of interconnectivity in the neighbourhood of player i, being defined as follows:

$$cc_i[t] = \frac{\sum_{j\neq i}\sum_{l\neq i, j} a_{ij}[t] a_{jl}[t] a_{ki}[t]}{\left(\sum_{j\neq i} a_{ij}[t]\right)^2 - \sum_{j\neq i}\left(a_{ij}[t]\right)^2} \tag{4.31}$$

such that $cc[t] = [cc_i[t]] \in R^{1 \times N}$ is the vector of the clustering coefficient of players. The higher the clustering coefficient of a player, the higher the cooperation between its teammates, meaning that if it tends to zero, the teammates do not cooperate much with each other. The relationship between the clustering coefficient and the connectivity has been used to describe structural (hierarchical) properties of networks (Ravasz & Barabási, 2003). By combining both metrics, it is possible to identify which players have a higher level of cooperation in terms of its positioning field established by the coach's strategy. For instance, midfielders and forwards are expected to have a higher degree of cooperation when compared to other positions (e.g., goalkeeper).

Global Rank

As stated, the relationship between the clustering coefficient and the connectivity can be used to describe the structural properties of networks. However, to do so, a weighting distribution between both should be taken into account, leading to the following weighting function, denoted as global rank:

$$g_i[t] = \rho_s s_i[t] + \rho_c c_i[t] \tag{4.32}$$

where $\rho_s + \rho_c = 1$, such that $g[t] = [g_i[t]] \in R^{1 \times N}$ is the vector of the global rank of players, with $0 \leq g_i \leq 1$. Taking into account that the main objective of players is to give priority to the collective performance (i.e., the overall interaction between players), one can ponder a balanced consideration of $\rho_s = \rho_c = 0.5$. The top-ranked player, i.e., the one presenting the higher $g_i[t]$, will then be denoted as the 'centroid player' (Horvath, 2011), which is calculated as follows:

$$i_c[t] = \underset{i}{\operatorname{argmax}} \, g_i[t] \tag{4.33}$$

Within football, the centroid player $i_c[t]$ could be considered as a hierarchically superior member (e.g., or key player). Note that $i_c[t]$ depends on t, meaning that the centroid player may change during a match. Moreover, if one considers two separated networks, one for passes performed and another for passes received, then it is likely that the key player for passes performed may be different from the key player for passes received.

Centroid Conformity

The network centroid, which is a result of $g_i[t]$ from Equation (4.35), defines the most centrally located player, i.e., the most highly connected node in the network. The connectivity strength between other players and the centroid player can be calculated as follows:

$$cc_{ii_c}[t] = \begin{cases} a_{i,\,i_c}[t],\, i \neq i_c \\ 1, i = i_c \end{cases} \qquad (4.34)$$

This inter-player analysis is denoted as centroid conformity and corresponds to the adjacency between the centroid player $i_c[t]$ and the ith player, such that $cc[t] = [cc_i[t]] \in R^{1 \times N}$ is the vector of the centroid conformity of players. In other words, $cc_{ii_c}[t]$ presents the cooperation level of the ith player with the top-ranked player.

Topological (Inter)dependency

The inter-player network analysis is based on the topological overlap presented in several works, such as Ravasz et al. (2003) and Horvath (2011), which represents the pair of players who cooperates with the same players. This measure also represents the overlap between two players even if they do not directly cooperate with one another. In other words, the topological overlap between the ith player and the jth player depends on the number of interactions they share with the same players, but it does not take into account the number of interactions between them.

The topological overlap is represented by a symmetric matrix, thus presenting the overlap between players, but neglecting the most independent player of the pair. Therefore, by using the concepts inherent to the clustering coefficient (Equation 4.34), one should consider not only the 'shared' interactions but also the influence of the conjoint interactions among players i and j. In other words, if two players interact with the same other players, then the cooperation between both of them allows building triangular relations between the other players. However, the ith player may be more dependable from the jth player if the former only interacts with the same players than player jth who, in turn, is able to interact with other players.

As a result, similarly to Ravasz et al. (2003) and Horvath (2011), one can define a topological dependency $T_d[t] = \left[td_{ij}[t]\right] \in R^{n \times n}$ as follows:

$$td_{ij}[t] = \begin{cases} \dfrac{\sum_{l \neq i,\, j} a_{il}[t]\, a_{lj}[t]\, a_{ij}[t]}{\sum_{l \neq i} a_{il}[t]}, \, i < j \\[2em] \dfrac{\sum_{l \neq i,\, j} a_{il}[t]\, a_{lj}[t]\, a_{ij}[t]}{\sum_{l \neq j} a_{lj}[t]}, \, i > j \\[2em] 1, i = j \end{cases} \qquad (4.35)$$

with i, j, $l = 1,2,\ldots, N$. As a consequence, two players have a high topological dependency, i.e., $td_{ij}[t] = 1$, if they interact with the same players and with one another. In other words, the more players they 'share', the stronger their cooperation and they are more likely to represent a small cluster.

Since T_d corresponds to a square matrix with the size equal to the number of players and since that it is not symmetric, i.e., $td_{ij}[t] \neq td_{ji}[t]$, it makes it difficult to compare the $td_{ij}[t]$ and $td_{ji}[t]$ pairs (Clemente et al., 2014). Therefore, to complement the previous analysis, the **topological inter-dependency** $T_{id}[t] = \left[ti_{ij}[t] \right] \in R^{N \times N}$ has been introduced as follows:

$$T_{id}[t] = T_d[t] - T_d[t]^T \tag{4.36}$$

where $T_d[t]^T$ is the transpose of matrix $T_d[t]$ and $T_{id}[t]$ corresponds to an antisymmetric square matrix, i.e., $ti_{ij}[t] = -ti_{ji}[t]$. In football and other team sports, one can easily observe dependencies between players, such that if $ti_{ij}[t] > 0$, then the ith player depends on the jth player to cooperate with the remaining teammates. Moreover, when associated with other network analysis (e.g., centroid player), the relative topological dependency allows identifying possible dependencies between players and even hierarchical relations (Clemente et al., 2014).

Density

The player connectivity calculated in Equation (4.24) allows retrieving several other team network analyses, such as the network density, which can be defined as follows:

$$D(t) = 2 \frac{\sum_{i \neq j}^{N} a_{ij}[t]}{N(N-1)} \tag{4.37}$$

Within players' networks, the density measures the overall cooperation among athletes. A density that tends to 1 indicates that all players strongly interact with each other.

Heterogeneity

Another network analysis based on the connectivity of players is the network heterogeneity, which is closely related to the variation of connectivity across players (Albert, Jeong, & Barabási, 2000; Watts, 2002), defined as the coefficient of variation of the connectivity distribution:

$$H(t) = \sqrt{\frac{N \sum c_i[t]^2 - \left(\sum c_i[t]\right)^2}{\left(\sum c_i[t]\right)^2}} \qquad (4.38)$$

Since the heterogeneity is invariant with respect to multiplying the connectivity by a scalar, one could use the scaled connectivity instead. Many complex networks have been found to exhibit an approximate scale-free topology, which implies that these networks are very heterogeneous. In other words, a high heterogeneity of the football network means that the players exhibit a high level of performance and there is, collectively, a low level of cooperation between players (Clemente et al., 2014).

Centralization

The network centrality, or degree centralization as Freeman (1978) addresses, can be defined as follows:

$$C = \frac{N}{N-2}\left(\frac{\max_{i \neq j} a_{ij}[t]}{N-1} - D\right) \qquad (4.39)$$

A centralization close to 1 means that one player strongly cooperates with all other players who, in turn, present a small (or inexistent) cooperation with each other. In contrast, a centralization of 0 indicates that all players cooperate equally among each other.

Conclusion

This chapter summarized and mathematically defined a series of computational metrics proposed over the past years to model the athletic performance of athletes and teams. These metrics are described on a feature-engineering perspective, to be seen as measurable properties of sport performance and to feed AI approaches for pattern recognition (Nargesian et al., 2017). The presented feature selection has been achieved through the close collaboration between sport scientists, engineers, and mathematicians, many of whom share the authorship of this book.

It is expected that, in a near future, feature engineering shall be accomplished in a more automated manner, leading to major breakthroughs in artificial intelligence for performance analysis in sports. This would allow practitioners to automatically extract the most relevant and representative features without direct human input, additionally tackling the 'curse of dimensionality' by reducing the number of features, as already achieved in other domains (Tang, Kay, & He, 2016). Deep learning algorithms are paving the way into the automated extraction of complex data representations at high levels of abstraction. They inherently provide a layered, hierarchical architecture of learning and data representation, where higher-level (more abstract) features are defined in terms of lower-level (less abstract) features.

Notes

1 https://www.mathworks.com/matlabcentral/fileexchange/69381-sample-entropy.
2 https://www.mathworks.com/matlabcentral/fileexchange/24035-wgplot-weighted-graph-plot-a-better-version-of-gplot.

5

ARTIFICIAL INTELLIGENCE FOR PATTERN RECOGNITION IN SPORTS

Classifying Actions and Performance Signatures

Introduction

Many have foreseen the adoption of artificial intelligence (AI) to solve complex problems, including those that cannot be solved by humans – at least not as efficiently as machines would (Russell & Norvig, 2002). However, the majority of the problems faced by mankind require the human expertise to lead and supervise the AI, being this latter used to complement, inform, and provide scale and depth to the understanding of such complex problems (Nilsson, 2014). AI has been employed in many domains worldwide, including marketing, agriculture, healthcare, gaming, robotics, and others, in such a way that the AI market is expected to represent a 200 billion euros industry by 2026 (Khillari, 2020). Some believe that this might lead to unemployment and an economic crisis never felt before (Ford, 2013), and others believe that it may solve the current crisis occurring in the healthcare sector (Meskó, Hetényi, & Győrffy, 2018), in our legal system (Berman & Hafner, 1989), and in many other critical pillars of mankind (Cortès, Sànchez-Marrè, Ceccaroni, R-Roda, & Poch, 2000). While several domains are overfilled with AI applications and related technologies, AI in sports is still in its infancy. Many sport scientists have discussed it over more than two decades ago (e.g., Lapham & Bartlett, 1995; McCarthy, 1997; Zelic, Kononenko, Lavrac, & Vuga, 1997), but its true potential has only been unleashed a few years ago, with the advent of new technologies, namely graphical processing units (GPUs), and powerful methods, including deep learning approaches (Liu, Yan, Liu, & Ma, 2017; Mora & Knottenbelt, 2017).

AI encompasses a wide range of tools developed with a strong mathematical foundation and developed to solve a wide range of different problems. Starting with the obvious, AI methods have been used to solve problems using logic-based approaches. Fuzzy set theory is perhaps the most widely adopted method, especially in control theory problems, assigning a degree of truth between 0 and 1 to vague statements to mimic the linguistic imprecision of human reasoning. Fuzzy logic has been also employed outside control theory problems, such as in decision-making architectures (Zimmermann, 2012), namely used as a warning system of disease outbreaks (Couceiro, Figueiredo, Luz, & Delorme, 2014). Going beyond logic, but still, in an attempt to mimic human reasoning, probability theory, and economics brought powerful tools over the past decades, such as Bayesian networks (Barber, 2012). Yet, this and other probabilistic methods have also been used for data mining procedures, including filtering, prediction, smoothing and others (Heckerman, 1997), and robotics (Ferreira & Dias, 2014).

Despite the relevance of logic-based and probabilistic-based methods in a wide panoply of problems, these methods often experience a combinatorial explosion, becoming exponentially slower as the problems grew larger (Russell & Norvig, 2003). This is the case for search and optimization problems. Search and optimization problems are, perhaps, the most common problem solved by AI. These methods can be used, for instance, to find the optimal path between a start and a target goal with minimal energy consumption and maximum gain. Simple exhaustive searches, i.e., non-AI, are rarely sufficient for most real-world problems due to the high dimensionality of the search space, known as 'the curse of dimensionality' (Bellman, 1966). The mathematical theory of optimization is, perhaps, one of the most efficient AI methods to solve these complex problems, starting the search with some form of a guess and then refining it incrementally until no more refinements can be made. Swarm intelligence, a particular case of AI, has been a subtype of optimization methods able to tackle most of the high-dimensionality problems based on biomimetics (Kennedy, 2006).

Solving optimization problems paves the way towards AI's end-goal into mimicking learning. Learning has been built in in many AI methods, ranging from classification to segmentation and in its many different forms and application domains. Generally, these AI methods use some sort of pattern matching to determine the closest match. The pattern to be recognized can either follow certain predefined classes delineated based on human expertise (supervised) or not (unsupervised). The latter follows the principles of self-organization, being often adopted to find unknown patterns in data or to find features, which can be useful for subsequent categorization. As this book adopts AI to augment human understanding of known behaviours, with well-studied performance patterns and established computational metrics (see Chapter 4), then the methods here addressed fall in the former.

In supervised learning, each pattern belongs to a certain predefined class, or label, which, within sports, can represent a different athlete, a performed action, or almost anything else needed to support the decision-making of coaches and technical teams. As stated in Chapter 4, the kinematic and physiological data typically acquired from the athletic performance is computed with the intent to extract relevant representative features. Sets of features are then labelled by human experts and stored as a dataset. The supervised learning methods are then trained based on the dataset to match a given cluster of data with its corresponding class (training phase). How this matching process is carried out highly depends on the supervised method adopted. However, regardless of the method, when new unknown raw data is received, a set of features is extracted out of it and fed into the trained method, which is then able to match it to an existing class based on its previous experience (testing phase).

All this general classification approach is better illustrated in Figure 5.1. The football kick is used as a practical example, from which kinematic data, more specifically the angular velocity, is extracted from the thigh and lower kicking

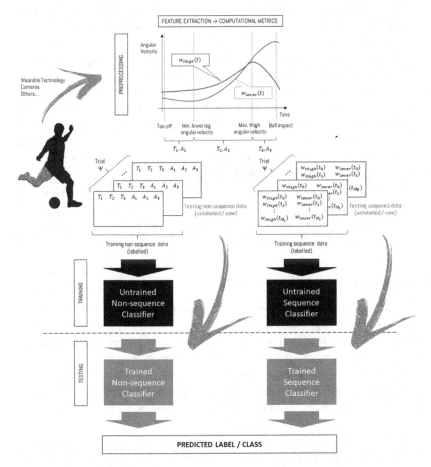

FIGURE 5.1   General classification approach applied to the football kick.

leg (Nunome, Ikegami, Kozakai, Apriantono, & Sano, 2006a; Nunome, Lake, Georgakis, & Stergioulas, 2006b). Raw data may or may not be pre-processed by adopting data cleaning, data transformation, and data reduction approaches (García, Luengo, & Herrera, 2016). Afterwards, feature extraction takes place by employing computational metrics, such as the ones presented in Chapter 4. Generally, and for most classification problems, the size of the set of features is known a priori as these are not time-dependent. Put it differently, and within sports context, a given set of features, with a known dimension, can be computed out of a time series, such as kinematic and physiological data or even time-dependent computational metrics, independent of the number of samples acquired. This is the typical classification problem, here identified as **non-sequence classification** to better distinguish it from the alternative, which can be dealt with a wide range of traditional approaches. In Figure 5.1, this set of 'static' features is represented by $\text{Ж} = \{T_i, A_i\}$ with $i = \{1,2,3\}$, which can represent the duration and the amplitude of the angular velocity (e.g., minimum lower leg angular velocity), being then extracted from the time series (angular velocities of thigh and lower kicking leg). Nevertheless, whenever time-dependent features are considered, as the ones previously extracted out of the computational metrics presented in Chapter 4, then **sequence classification** needs to be taken into account. In Figure 5.1, this set of dynamic features is represented by the angular velocity of the thigh $w_{thigh}(t)$ and the angular velocity of the lower leg $w_{lower}(t)$, thus leading to a two-dimensional input feature data, $\text{Ж}(t) = \{w_{thigh}(t), w_{lower}(t)\}$, with a variable sequence length. Regardless of the approach, a large labelled dataset is often used for training and, after the classifier is trained, it shall then be able to autonomously predict the label/class inherent to new incoming data.

The following sections describe both **non-sequence classification** and **sequence classification**, what they intend to tackle more specifically in sports, and present some of the most widely used methods adopted in the literature.

Non-Sequence Classification

A non-sequence classifier, commonly known as traditional classifier, adopts machine learning approaches to classify a set of features of a known size. For instance, for facial recognition software, this set of features may include the typical facial features, such as the relative position, size, and/or shape of the eyes, nose, cheekbones, and jaw (Brunelli & Poggio, 1993). For speech emotion recognition, features such as pitch, timing, voice quality, and articulation are often adopted. In sports, as in other human movement analysis domains, this set of features is often calculated based on certain time series (e.g., kinematics). For instance, for gait analysis, the set of features can be based on non-time–dependent variables, such as the height of an individual, but some of the features can also be computed based on time-dependent kinematical data, such as the amount of bounce of the whole body in a full stride, the side-to-side sway of the torso, the maximum distance between the front and the back legs at the peak of the swing phase of a stride, and the amount of arm and leg swing, among others (Lee & Grimson, 2002). Put it differently, a set of features of a known size can have, as input, a set of time series of an unknown size, which depend on the duration of a given movement. Figure 5.1 previously presented depicts such example, where a set of 'static' features (duration and amplitude $\mathfrak{K} = \{T_i, A_i\}$ with $i = \{1,2,3\}$ are extracted from a given task execution (football kick).

The main advantage of non-sequence classification over its sequential counterpart is then obvious: fewer data used as input. Each feature is represented by a single value, often a real number, i.e., $\in R^1$, and while many can be used within the same set, the amount of data being fed to the classifier is considerably smaller than in sequence classification. For instance, in the example presented in Figure 5.1, each one-dimensional time series $w_{thigh}(t)$ and $w_{lower}(t)$ comprise many real numbers $\in R^1$ – one for each timestamp t. Meaning that, if the football kick lasts around 40 ms and the data acquisition equipment (e.g., camera) offers a sampling rate of 200 Hz (Nunome et al., 2006a, 2006b), then instead of 16 samples (8 for each $w_{thigh}(t)$ and $w_{lower}(t)$), the classifier would encompass only the six features T_i, A_i with $i = \{1,2,3\}$. This also implies that the number of features for non-sequence classifiers remains the same, regardless of the duration of the movement. Put it differently, the computational complexity of a given non-sequence classifier will remain the same for a certain number of features and classes, which remains unchanged within the same dataset.

Their intrinsic simplicity and computational complexity, when compared to sequence classification, makes traditional methods to be widely adopted under many domains. However, their performance greatly depends on the characteristics of the data, such as the dataset size, distribution of samples across classes, the dimensionality, and the noise. The decision tree is perhaps one of the most widely used machine learning algorithm (Safavian & Landgrebe, 1991). Other widely used classifiers are the Gaussian mixture model (Reynolds, 2009), the k-nearest neighbour algorithm (Cunningham & Delany, 2020), and the naïve Bayes classifier (Rish, 2001). All these methods have been widely adopted in sports-related problems, but the kernel-based support vector machine (SVM) and artificial neural network (ANN) methods are the most popular in the sport community (see Chapter 2). For their wide adoption when no matching model is available and considering accuracy over speed or scalability, SVM and ANN are further described in the next sections.

Support Vector Machine

The support vector machine (SVM) is a classical machine learning technique employed to solve either linear or non-linear classification, as well as regression problems. The SVM was developed by Vladimir Vapnik with the intent to implement principles based on statistical learning theory (Hearst, Dumais, Osuna, Platt, & Scholkopf, 1998). The main objective of this method is to find the best hyperplane, in a D-dimensional space, capable of maximizing the margin between support vectors, i.e., different data classes near to the hyperplane. The distance between the support vectors is called margin which can be soft or hard, depending on whether the problem is linearly or non-linearly separable, respectively (Byvatov, Fechner, Sadowski, & Schneider, 2003).

Let us consider a dataset with heart rate data from two athletes while performing a given task, where the objective is to distinguish to whom that data belongs, i.e., if the heart rate data received comes from athlete one or two. Figure 5.2 depicts this one-dimensional problem (single feature/variable), where both classes, athlete one (blue) and two (green), are linearly separable. In this case, the SVM model would be able to easily classify the data since it is easy to find a point separating both clusters of data.

Nevertheless, most real-world problems are non-linear, i.e., they are not linearly separable. Therefore, for these cases, the idea is to adopt a linear separation by first mapping the data to a higher dimension using a non-linear function. Put it differently, a simple problem can be remapped to a more complex problem to be linearly separable. While it may sound like a paradox, this approach can easily be justified. For example, let us consider adopting a polynomial function to remap new heart rate data represented in Figure 5.3a, thus leading to Figure 5.3b. It is possible to observe that it would be impossible to linearly separate the original data since athlete two (green) had heart rate data in-between the heart rate data from athlete one (blue). However, by remapping it to a polynomial domain, the data can be easily clustered using a straight line modelled by a linear equation. This implies that a hyperplane has been created by mapping the data to a higher dimension, where it is possible to easily separate the two different classes, previously inseparable in their original plane.

Mapping the input data, or features, is done by using the support vectors as a part of the training data, influencing the decision according to similarities between new points. Due to the complexity of these problems and to map accordingly, a kernel function is used, incorporating the a priori knowledge (Ben-Hur & Weston, 2010). That is, for non-linear SVM problems, mapping the training data, here denoted as X_{data}, from the input space Φ to a high-dimensional feature space χ, is required:

$$\Phi : X_{data} \rightarrow \chi \tag{5.1}$$

FIGURE 5.2 Linear separable data (adapted from Manning, Raghavan, & Schütze, 2008).

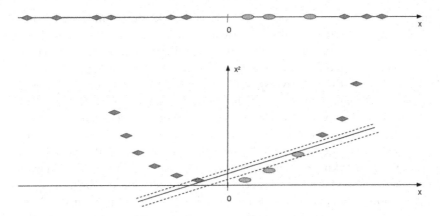

FIGURE 5.3 Non-linear separable data (adapted from Manning et al., 2008).

The kernel function, K, then calculates the inner product of the vectors (x_p, y_p) belonging to the feature space, as can be seen in the below equation:

$$K(x_p, y_p) = \Phi(x_p) \cdot \Phi(y_p) \tag{5.2}$$

Schölkopf (2001) observed that the kernel function can define a distance, d_{kernel}, on the input space as follows:

$$d_{kernel}^{2(x_p, y_p)} = \left(\Phi(x_p) \cdot \Phi(y_p)\right)^2 = K(x_p, y_p) - 2K(x_p, y_p) + K(y_p, y_p) \tag{5.3}$$

This shows that the kernel function, $K(x_p, y_p)$, can be described as a degree of similarity between the samples x_p and y_p. In practice, there are plenty of kernel functions to be adopted, being the polynomial, Gaussian, and sigmoidal the most common (Lorena & de Carvalho, 2007). In the example from Figure 5.3, the kernel function adopted to map the data was a polynomial function, being mathematically described as follows:

$$K(x_p, y_p) = \left(x_p \cdot y_p + c_p\right)^q \tag{5.4}$$

where q is the order of the kernel and c_p is a free parameter which influences higher-order versus lower-order terms in the polynomial equation.

Neural Network

Artificial neural networks (ANNs), often known simply as neural network, are mathematical or computational models designed based on the human central nervous system. An ANN is based on the synapse processes that occur in our brain. An ANN is composed of several nuclei that connect each other creating several relationships as a network of several artificial neurons (Brumatti, 2005). The artificial neuron is a logical and mathematical structure with behaviour and functions similar to a biological neuron (Graupe, 2007). The analogy with collective sports is inevitable since the interconnection between the neurons of an ANN happens in different layers. In a football game, the ball moves from player to player until the objective is accomplished. In a rather simplistic manner, during the offensive phase, the objective is reached if a goal is scored. As the ball approaches the goal, several layers are conquered, taking into account that, sometimes, it is necessary to retreat or remain in one layer for a longer period to understand the weaknesses of the opposing team and delineate a more effective offensive play. In an ANN, the first layer consists of the input neurons, or features, which, through the synapses, they send data to the second layer and so on, until it reaches the last layer of neurons, which outputs the result (Yadav, Yadav, & Jain, 2014). Synapses store the transition parameters between each layer, called 'weights', and it should be noted that the more complex the system, the more layers it shall have (Priddy, 2005).

An ANN is defined by three levels (Kumar & Sharma, 2014):

1   Model of interconnection between the different levels of neurons;
2   Learning process to update the weights of the interconnections;
3   The activation function that converts input into output.

As far as the learning process of ANNs is concerned, it can be both supervised and non-supervised (Li, 1994). As previously stated, supervised learning is where this book falls in, which, for an ANN, relies on the presence of an external agent who checks how close the results are from reality (from training data), changing the weights between the neurons in order to make the classification more efficient. This shows that the weights are the main responsible for memorizing patterns and making decisions. In non-supervised learning, while not addressed here, it is interesting to highlight that there is no a priori knowledge of network outputs, so it does not make use of an external agent. Therefore, the network distinguishes classes with different patterns through learning algorithms based on neighbourhood and grouping concepts. In this case, the network is adjusted according to the statistical regularities of the input data.

To better illustrate these concepts, let us consider a neural network that aims to determine whether an offensive play was a success ($y_{out} = 1$) or not ($y_{out} = -1$), considering a binary input dataset $\left(x_{inp1}, x_{inp2}, x_{inp3}\right)$ containing the sequence of passes between three players, respectively, being that 1 represents the involvement of the player in the sequence. This type of linear (binary) single-layer ANN, known as perceptron, is illustrated in Figure 5.4.

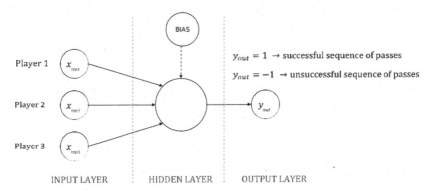

FIGURE 5.4 Illustration of a single-layer neural network.

Learning starts by feeding the model. Let $\mathcal{K} = \{x_{inp1}, x_{inp2}, x_{inp3}\}$ be the input data. Consider that the following sequences have been studied beforehand and, therefore, used to train the model (as references):

1 $\left(x_{inp1}, x_{inp2}, x_{inp3}\right) = (0,0,1),\ y_{out} = -1$
2 $\left(x_{inp1}, x_{inp2}, x_{inp3}\right) = (1,1,0),\ y_{out} = 1$

The initial weights were randomly defined as $w_1 = 0.4$, $w_2 = -0.6$, and $w_3 = 0.6$, the bias as $w_0 = 0.5$, and the learning rate as $\eta = 0.4$.

At each step of the algorithm, a new y_{out} needs to be calculated, renamed as y_{out}^{calc} for the sake of simplicity. During training, the weights are then systematically updated until this new y_{out}^{calc} matches the ground truth y_{out} labelled/defined by the designer (e.g., coach who assessed a given sequence of passes as successful or unsuccessful). To calculate y_{out}^{calc}, the weights are multiplied by their respective input as follows:

$$y_{out}^{calc} = \begin{cases} \sum x_{inpk} w_k w_0 \\ \\ \sum x_{inpk} w_k w_0 \end{cases} \tag{5.5}$$

For instance, for the input $(0,0,1)$, which means that only player 3 participated in the offensive play, whose expected output is $y_{out} = -1$, the calculated output is $y_{out}^{calc} = 1$, since $0 \times (0.4) + 0 \times (-0.6) + 1 \times (0.6) - 1 \times (0.5) = 0.1 > 0$. This means that the calculated output, y_{out}^{calc}, does not match the output provided by the designer for that known sequence, y_{out}, thus meaning that the hyperplane is unable to separate the two classes properly, as depicted in Figure 5.5a.

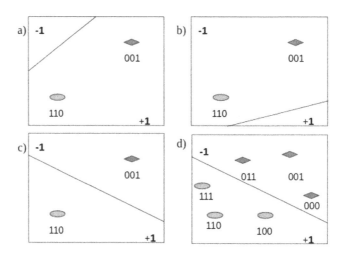

FIGURE 5.5 Network's output: (a) after the first training step, (b) after the second training step, (c) after the third training step, (d) after using new sequences (testing).

Therefore, since $y_{out}^{calc} \neq y_{out}$, one needs to update the weights until this condition is verified. The generic form for changing weights, by error correction, is defined by the follow equation:

$$w_k = w_k + \eta e x_{inpk} \tag{5.6}$$

where η is the learning rate and x_{inpk} represents the input of the neuron k at a given instant. The weight for the next iteration is always calculated with respect to the current weight value w_k. The term e represents the error which is given by (Cintra, Velho, & Todling, 2011; Jain, Mao, & Mohiuddin, 1996) the following equation:

$$e = y_{out} - y_{out}^{calc} \tag{5.7}$$

By adopting these equations, this leads to $w_1 = 0.4 + 0.4 \times (-1 - (+1)) \times (0) = 0.4$, $w_2 = -0.6 + 0.4 \times (-1 - (+1)) \times (0) = -0.6$, $w_3 = 0.6 + 0.4 \times (-1 - (+1)) \times (1) = -0.2$, and $w_0 = 0.5 + 0.4 \times (-1 - (+1)) \times (-1) = 1.3$. This is followed by testing these new weights for the next input value $(1,1,0)$, representing a sequence where players 1 and 2 participate. Again, while the expected output is $y_{out} = 1$, the calculated output is $y_{out}^{calc} = -1$, since $1 \times (0.4) + 1 \times (-0.6) + 0 \times (-0.2) - 1 \times (1.3) = -1.5 \leq 0$. As $y_{out}^{calc} \neq y_{out}$, the weights need to be, once again, updated, leading to $w_1 = 1.2$, $w_2 = 0.2$, $w_2 = -0.2$, and $w_0 = 0.5$ (Figure 5.5b).

Since the two sequences used for training have been evaluated, a second round takes place, starting again with input $(0,0,1)$. This time, and with the newly found weights, $y_{out}^{calc} = y_{out} = -1$, since $0 \times (1.2) + 0 \times (0.2) + 1 \times (-0.2) - 1 \times (0.5)$. $= -0.7 \leq 0$ Since this condition is now verified and the desired response matches the response provided by the ANN, there is no need to update the weights. Likewise, for the second input sequence, $(1,1,0)$, $y_{out}^{calc} = y_{out} = 1$, since $1 \times (1.2) + 1 \times (0.2) + 0 \times (-0.2) - 1 \times (0.5) = 0.9 > 0$, proving that these weights allow the model to correctly classify both sequences of passes as successful and unsuccessful (Figure 5.5c).

While still holding to this very simplistic example, let us now suppose that new sequences have been acquired, namely:

1 $\left(x_{inp1}, x_{inp2}, x_{inp3} \right) = (0,0,0), y_{out} = ?$
2 $\left(x_{inp1}, x_{inp2}, x_{inp3} \right) = (1,1,1), y_{out} = ?$
3 $\left(x_{inp1}, x_{inp2}, x_{inp3} \right) = (1,0,0), y_{out} = ?$
4 $\left(x_{inp1}, x_{inp2}, x_{inp3} \right) = (0,1,1), y_{out} = ?$

What would then be the expected output for each of these sequences involving different interactions from players 1, 2, and 3? It shall be obvious that in the first case, where players have not collaborated at all for the sequence (so the sequence does not even exist in the first place), it should lead to an unsuccessful sequence. Maybe it could be also obvious, to some extent, that the second sequence involving all the players would be treated as successful, considering that players 1 and 2 were already able to establish a successful sequence before. For the third and fourth sequences, however, the rationale may not be as straightforward.

To assess the performance of the basic ANN previously presented and considering that it was trained with only two sequences, let us now feed the network with these new untested data. For input $(0,0,0)$, $y_{out}^{calc} = -1$, since $0 \times (1.2) + 0 \times (0.2) + 0 \times (-0.2) - 1 \times (0.5) = -0.5 \leq 0$, meaning that a sequence where players do not participate in (which is not even an offensive sequence in the first place) is unsurprisingly classified as unsuccessful. For input $(1,1,1)$, $y_{out}^{calc} = 1$, since $1 \times (1.2) + 1 \times (0.2) + 1 \times (-0.2) - 1 \times (0.5) = 0.7 > 0$, meaning that a sequence where all the players participate in is classified as successful, being in line with the rationale previously established. As for input $(1,0,0)$, $y_{out}^{calc} = 1$, since $1 \times (1.2) + 0 \times (0.2) + 0 \times (-0.2) - 1 \times (0.5) = 0.7 > 0$, meaning that a sequence where only player 1 participates is classified as successful. However, for input $(0,1,1)$, $y_{out}^{calc} = -1$, since $0 \times (1.2) + 1 \times (0.2) + 1 \times (-0.2) - 1 \times (0.5) = -0.5 \leq 0$, meaning that a sequence where players 2 and 3 collaborate, but without player 1, is classified as unsuccessful.

Even though this is a very simplistic example, mostly adopted for the sake of explaining how a linear (binary) single-layer ANN works, it shows that the way the ANN makes a decision (classifies) is aligned, in a way, with how humans would do. It is noteworthy that this ANN has been trained with only two sequences, which is far from unrealistic, and still allows us to conclude that player 1, for the above examples, is key in establishing successful offensive plays.

Sequence Classification

Sequence classification is a modelling problem in which the input data is dynamic. Data is time-variant, using sequences over space or time as inputs, and sequence classification, just as non-sequence classification, intends to classify the category where that data fits in. Sequence data can be characterized as a sequence of item sets that represents the behaviour of, for example, a player over a specific period or task. Contrarily to non-sequence classifiers, which typically classify features of a known size, sequence classification works with sequential data of unknown and variant size, as it is the example of the daily values of a currency exchange rate, the acoustic features at successive time stamps for speech recognition, or classifies whether a patient is healthy by analysing ECG time-series data within healthcare settings (Bishop, 2006; Xing, Pei, & Keogh, 2010).

Within sports, and as already mentioned in the previous section, there are many applications where the set of features are often time-based. In the example from Figure 5.1, both 'static' and 'time-variant' features can be extracted from a football kick. The sequence data in Figure 5.1 comprises the angular velocity of the thigh $w_{thigh}(t)$ and the angular velocity of the lower leg $w_{lower}(t)$, $Ж(t) = \{w_{thigh}(t), w_{lower}(t)\}$. As expected, this leads to a variable sequence length even when using the same setup, since a penalty kick may not always have the same duration and, therefore, $Ж$ in trial 1 ($\Psi = 1$) is likely to have a different dimension in trial 2 ($\Psi = 2$).

In sequence classification models, the current output depends on the previous input throughout the entire dataset. Considering this general dependence on past observations, it would be impractical for the model to process all the information due to the increasing complexity required. To tackle that, machine learning methods, as ensemble learning and deep learning methods, have been proposed.

Ensemble Learning

Most of the classification methods perform their function based on the probabilities resulting from their output. In order to increase the overall classification performance (bias), and decrease the variance, the probabilistic combination of different classifiers has been widely explored by the community, giving rise to the term 'ensemble learning'. The classifiers chosen to be part of this ensemble system have to meet some conditions as classifiers with low bias tend to have a high variance. However, by averaging the results, it will reduce the variance and thus increase the probability of correct classification. Ensemble systems have received some attention due to its versatility to solve a different kind of real-world applications problems. To better understand this concept, one can consider that a decision made by an ensemble-based system is no more than a decision made by a human being, i.e., whenever we need to make an important decision, we tend to seek for other's opinions so we can build our own and reach a more confident decision (Polikar, 2012).

Ensemble classification methods can be sequential or parallel. In sequential classification, the base learners are generated sequentially aiming to make the most of the dependencies between models. Within parallel ensemble methods, the models are generated in parallel, i.e., it encourages the independence between the base learners and, consequently, it reduces the error by averaging the output from the multiple models. Ensemble classification methods can also be homogeneous, using the same type of base learners, or heterogeneous, where base learners are different from each other (Zhou, 2012).

This section describes the dynamic Bayesian mixture model (DBMM) ensemble classifier, which benefits from the concept of dynamically mixing classifiers by combining the conditional probabilities resulting from each different classifier in order to have the best possible result. Throughout the classification process in DBMM, a weight is assigned to each classifier according to the previous knowledge resulting from the training process. This weight acts as the level of confidence that is placed on the respective classifiers, being updated during the classification process. At each moment t, the set of classifiers considers the Bayesian probability as a mean to assess the contribution from each classifier to the result. The result of this ensemble model is presented as a weighted sum of the distributions, combining the results of the different models in a single one.

Assuming that $Ж$ represents the input data of the base learners and that the output of all of the base learners contains the class prediction, those results are then combined and stored in $y_{out}^{comb}(t)$, for each time step t, forming $Ж$ that is the input data for DBMM, for the same time t. Thus, DBMM corresponds to the set of classification models represented by $Ж(t) = \left\{ y_{out}^{comb}(1),\ y_{out}^{comb}(2),\ \ldots,\ y_{out}^{comb}(t) \right\}$. The DBMM resulting probability is then given by the following equation:

$$P\big(C(t)|Ж\big) = \beta \times M_{trans} \times \sum_{d=1}^{CL} w_d(t) \times P_d\big(Ж|\,C(t)\big) \tag{5.8}$$

where $\beta = \dfrac{1}{\sum jP\big(C_j(t)|\,C_j(t-1)\big) \times \sum_{i=1}^{N} w_i(t) \times P_d\big(Ж|\,C_j(t)\big)}$ is the normal-

ization factor, necessary due to the continuous updating of the confidence level, and j is the index for the set of posteriors of a certain base learner d. M_{trans} is the model for the probability of state transition between class variables, or states, over time. This model can represent the *a priori* in the DBMM, as a dynamic probabilistic cycle, where the current *posteriori* becomes the new *a priori*. The weight $w_d(t)$ for each time frame t is estimated through the level of confidence based on entropy. The $P_d(\text{Ж} \mid C(t))$ is the *a posteriori* result for the base classifier cl in t, which becomes the probability of the mixing model, with $cl = \{1,\ldots, CL\}$ – CL being the total number of classifiers considered in the model. It should be noted that when normalization is applied, the class C at time t is conditioned to the class obtained at time $t-1$. This describes a non-stationary behaviour, where the posterior of the previous time of each class becomes the current *prior* for the classification at time t.

As already mentioned, a confidence level is assigned to each classifier by using a weight calculated based on the entropy of each basic classifier, $En_d(L)$, through the analysis of the later probabilities previously observed:

$$En_d(L) = -\sum L_j \times \log(L_j) \tag{5.9}$$

where L_j represents a set with conditional probabilities $P_d(C(t)\mid \text{Ж})$ given by the base classifier $cl = \{1,\ldots, CL\}$ and j is the index for the set of posteriors of a specific base classifier cl. After knowing En_d, the weight $w_d(t)$ for each base classifier is obtained in two steps, being necessary, in a first step, to calculate the global value of the weight:

$$\forall w_d, \ w_d(t) = \left[1 - \left(\frac{En_d}{\displaystyle\sum_{d=1}^{CL} En_d} \right) \right] \tag{5.10}$$

where $En_d \equiv En_d(L)$ is the current entropy value. The second step is to normalize the weight:

$$w_d(t) = \frac{w_d(t)}{\displaystyle\sum_{d=1}^{CL} w_d(t)} \tag{5.11}$$

In order to make a local update of the weights and ensure a superior conviction, it is assumed that the system has a Markov-based memory during the online classification, obtaining temporal information from the set of posterior for each base classifier as $L_{\{d\ldots CL\}} = \{P(C_d(t)\mid C_d(t-1)); \ldots P(C_d(t-CL)\mid C_d(t-(CL-1)))\}$. This is combined with the weights at the time $t-1$, $w_d(t-1)$, to update the weights of each base classifier cl in the classification of each frame, as follows:

$$w_d(t) = \frac{w_d(t-1) \times P(w_{d_{new}} \mid En_d(L))}{\displaystyle\sum_{d=1}^{CL} w_d(t-1) \times P(w_{d_{new}} \mid En_d(L))} \tag{5.12}$$

where $w_{cl}(t)$ is the estimated weight that is updated by each base classifier at each instant of time and $w_{cl}(t-1)$ is given by the previous weight calculated at $t-1$. All of these concepts are illustrated in Figure 5.6, using the same passing sequence example described earlier in this chapter.

Consider the same example given in the previous 'Neural network' section, whose objective was to determine whether an offensive play was a success ($y_{out}=1$) or not ($y_{out}=-1$), considering an input dataset collected at 1 Hz, containing the sequence of passes between three players, respectively, being that 1 represents the involvement of the player in the sequence, and 0 his/her absence. First, the base learners used in the DBMM are chosen. If more than one base learner is chosen, the DBMM will, as a rule, provide a more robust solution since the base learners will use all of the available information to assess whether a given sequence is successful. Let us suppose that SVM and ANN (both described in the previous section) were chosen as base learners of the DBMM. Let us also consider the following sequences as input data for both base learners, at each time t, and the respective y_{out}:

$$1 \quad \left(x_{inp1}(t),\ x_{inp2}(t),\ x_{inp3}(t)\right) = \begin{bmatrix} 0 & 0 & 0 \\ 0 & 1 & 0 \\ 0 & 0 & 1 \end{bmatrix},\ y_{out}=-1$$

$$2 \quad \left(x_{inp1}(t),\ x_{inp2}(t),\ x_{inp3}(t)\right) = \begin{bmatrix} 1 & 1 & 0 \\ 1 & 0 & 0 \\ 1 & 0 & 1 \end{bmatrix},\ y_{out}=1$$

During training, the base learners output the probability a given set of features has to belong to a certain class which, in this case, is whether a given sequence

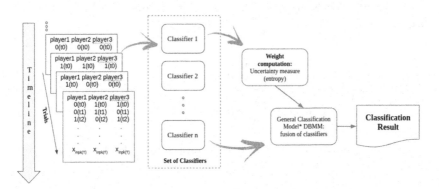

FIGURE 5.6   Illustrative representation of DBMM (adapted from Faria, Premebida, & Nunes, 2014).

of passes is either successful or unsuccessful. The DBMM is fed with results from both ANN ($cl = 1$) and SVM ($cl = 2$):

$$
Ж(t) = \begin{cases} y_{out}^{ANN} \\ y_{out}^{SVM} \end{cases}
$$

Based on the entropy of each base learner, the corresponding weight of each method is computed after each iteration. For the provided example, this could lead to $w_{d=1}(t) = 0.900$ and $w_{d=2}(t) = 0.100$. Before the weight value normalization, the predefined weight, randomly defined as $w_1(t-1) = 0.3500$ and $w_2(t-1) = 0.6500$ initially, is updated, for each base learner, by multiplying it with the entropy-based weight, leading to $w_1(t) = 0.900 \times 0.35 = 0.3150$ and $w_2(t) = 0.100 \times 0.65 = 0.0650$. To ensure that the sum of the weights is equal to 1, normalization is then needed. Adding both weights lead to a total weight of 0.3800, which, by applying Equation 5.11, leads to the normalized weight values $w_1(t) = 0.8289$ and $w_2(t) = 0.1711$.

These normalized weights allow the DBMM to dynamically infer the relevance of the classifiers over each step. For example, at time $t = 1$, the result of y_{out}^{DBMM} could be something like:

$$
y_{out}^{DBMM}(1) = \begin{cases} y_{out}^{ANN}(1) \times 0.8289 = \left[1.6175e^{-51}, 0.8289\right] \\ y_{out}^{SVM}(1) \times 0.1711 = [0.0757, 0.0954] \end{cases}
$$

Adding the values corresponding to the same class leads to:

$$
y_{out}^{DBMM}(1) = \begin{cases} 1.6175e^{-51} + 0.0757 = 0.0757 \\ 0.8289 + 0.0954 = 0.9243 \end{cases}
$$

Now multiplying it by the prior value, taking into account that the prior for the first input is $\dfrac{1}{CL}$, leads to:

$$
y_{out}^{DBMM}(1) = \begin{cases} 0.0757 \times \left(\dfrac{1}{2}\right) = 0.0378 \\ 0.9243 \times \left(\dfrac{1}{2}\right) = 0.4622 \end{cases}
$$

Dividing it by its sum allows us to find the probability value for each class as:

$$
y_{out}^{DBMM}(1) = \begin{cases} \dfrac{0.0378}{0.5} = 0.0757 \\ \dfrac{0.4622}{0.5} = 0.9243 \end{cases}
$$

Here we can see that, for the first test input (0,0,0), DBMM unsurprisingly classified it as class 2, that is, as unsuccessful ($y_{out} = -1$). For the next input (0,1,0), a similar process will be used to generate data from the model, excepting that, from now on, each decision is dependent on the decision taken at the previous time step. That is, at time $t = 2$, we first have to multiply the result of each of the base learners by the current normalized weight value (previously calculated) so that we can then compute the weighted sum for each class. Afterwards, we calculate the probability of the state transition between classes using priors, i.e., by multiplying the output at time by the current weight value. The last step is to normalize those values. This process is then repeated throughout the entire dataset, and as the inference process moves forward from the current time step (t) to the next ($t+1$), the oldest time step ($t-1$) is dropped off the network.

The main difference between this model and ANN might be unnoticeable in the first instance. However, the traditional ANN works generally well for static data. The complexity of the problem grows when using sequential data, which might prove itself to be extremely difficult for a single neural network to work with. By using ensembles, nonetheless, one relies not only on one model's output but in the combination of more than one output. If three anti-correlated base learners are chosen and one of the networks makes a mistake classifying one of the trials, the other two networks can still fix the error. There are, however, other types of neural networks able to deal with sequence data classification elegantly, as is the case of recurrent neural networks.

Recurrent Neural Network

A recurrent neural network (RNN) is a type of neural network where the output from the previous cell is the input for the next. This is possible due to their intrinsic loops, conceding the information to persist (Agatonovic-Kustrin $t = 1$ & Beresford, 2000). Put it differently, the RNN can be seen as multiple copies of the same network where the output from the first structure passes to the next, and so on until it reaches the last network structure. The RNN consists of an input layer, a hidden layer with recurrent connections responsible for the signal propagation, and the output layer $y_{out}(t)$. The input vector $\mathbb{K}(t)$ represents the data fed to the model and the output at the same time t. The decision made by an RNN at time $t-1$ is stored in the hidden layer, which then affects the decision at time t. This process allows the sequential information to be spread for many time steps. For supervised learning, the input vectors feed the network one vector at a time. Then, the result is calculated at each time step as a non-linear function containing the weighted sum of all connected units.

As in any ANN, the basis about training RNN remains similar. First, the input features go forward to the network and output the result. Then, that result is compared with the ground-truth label assessing the network's performance using a loss function. Lastly, and this is where the RNN differs from the traditional

ANN, the gradients for each structure are calculated based on the error value which will later update the weights through a backpropagation process, i.e., from the output to the inputs. The gradient values are used to adjust the weights, where a large gradient value means large weight adjustments and vice versa. As it backpropagates, all the gradients are calculated with respect to the previous, which may lead to some issues. When the gradient value from the previous layer is small, the gradient from the current layer will be even smaller, reducing the adjustments made on the weights and, consequently, failing to learn (Agatonovic-Kustrin & Beresford, 2000; Lipton, Berkowitz, & Elkan, 2015).

The process of carrying memory forward is modelled with the following equation:

$$h(t) = \sigma\left(W \star \mathbb{K}(t) + U \star h(t-1)\right) \tag{5.13}$$

where $h(t)$ is the hidden state at timestamp t and $\mathbb{K}(t)$ is the set of input features at the same time t. W is the weight's matrix and U represents the hidden-state-to-hidden-state matrix, which is also known as transition matrix. Summing up, the RNN decides upon two inputs, the recent past and the present, allowing the model to have memory in which the information that has passed through the structures is recalled. With this, it is possible to keep the information from the previous network state allowing performing temporal processing. Here, the output is no longer the result of the input signal, but a combination of that with the value of the previous state. Nevertheless, a precise prediction needs context. For example, the lack of context in these situations grows a gap between the relevant information and the point where that information is needed. The greater the gap, the more the RNN struggles to adequately connect information, leading to an inability to deal with long-term dependencies.

In a practical manner, let us consider that an RNN model needs to be trained to classify whether the player is attacking, defending, or counter-attacking. The model input data $\mathbb{K}(t)$ will contain three time-varying features, namely the Cartesian position in x and y, and the side of the field that the player is in (1 if the player is in its defensive half and −1 if it is in the offensive half). The model will learn the patterns of each of those tasks and, when feeding it, the model should be able to classify it as attacking, defending, and counter-attacking. For example, considering a player moving towards the opponent goal, by the variation of the positions x and y, and the side of the field, the model will learn that the player is attacking. However, a counter-attack is a play that involves more time and, consequently, a larger time-series sequence. That happens because, while in counter-attack, the model has to consider, first, the defence phase and, second, the attack phase. In that case, due to RNN's vanishing problem (Figure 5.7), the information that will be retained may as well only take into account the most recent information from the sequence, i.e., the attack.

In Figure 5.7, the darker circles represent a larger sensitivity. For the RNN (top) the sensitivity decays over time as new inputs overwrite the activation of hidden units and, consequently, the network forgets the first inputs. In other words, the larger the input (i.e., larger sequences), the larger the steps that RNN has to process, being unable to remember all past information. The RNN remembers things only for a limited period, and if a large amount of information is fed to the network, it will get lost somewhere. This is the known vanishing gradient problem or short-term memory problem of RNN (Graves & Schmidhuber, 2005; Schuster & Paliwal, 1997). There is, however, a particular type of RNN with an improved capability of learning long-term dependencies, known as Long Short-Term Memory (LSTM) networks.

LSTM tackles the issue of dealing with long-term dependencies by integrating information over long periods, which represents an important evolution, as it avoids the long-term dependency problem of the traditional RNN (Sak, Senior, & Beaufays, 2014), as can be seen at the bottom part of Figure 5.7. As

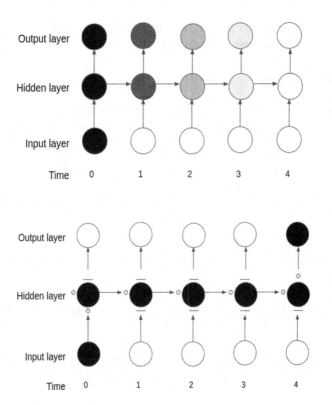

FIGURE 5.7 (Top) RNN vanishing problem (adapted from Nayel & Shashrekha, 2019), (bottom) preservation of information by LSTM (adapted from Graves, 2012).

in the top part, the dark nodes indicate the sensitivity of the node to the input information. Unlike it, however, LSTM comprises additional gates. The small circle represents an open gate and the horizontal line a closed gate. The input gate is represented below the node, to the left the forget gate, and the output gate rests above the hidden layer. The bottom part of Figure 5.7 exemplifies a case where the memory cell remembers the first input, while the forget gate is open and the input gate is closed. As presented in Figure 5.8, each LSTM cell has three major interacting gate layers: the forget gate, the memory gate, and the output gate. These 'special' gates are different tensor operations that can learn which information to add or remove from the hidden state, making short-term memory to be less of an issue. That is, the information is forwarded from the current neuron to the next neuron and so on throughout all the hidden layers. The first step begins in the sigmoid layer, known as the forget gate layer, $fg(t)$, where it is decided whether the previous information should be considered. The forget gate layer looks at the previous timestamp output, $h(t-1)$, and the new input, $Ж(t)$, and outputs a number between 0 and 1 for each number on the cell state $Cs(t-1)$.

Let us consider a certain instant t, the neuron input $Ж(t)$, and the output $h(t)$. The forget gate layer at instant t can be described as follows:

$$fg(t) = \sigma \left(W_{fg} \cdot \left[h(t-1),\ Ж(t) \right] + b_{fg} \right) \tag{5.14}$$

where σ is the sigmoid activation function, and W_{fg} and b_{fg} denote the weights and bias of the forget gate layer, respectively. The second step decides what new

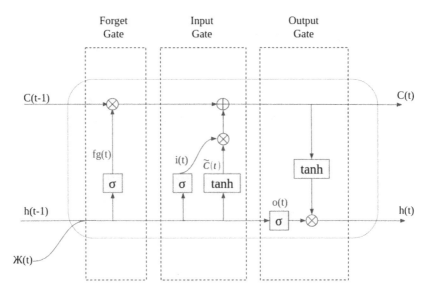

FIGURE 5.8 LSTM cell structure (adapted from Jiang et al., 2019).

information is going to be stored in the cell state. Here, a sigmoid layer, called the input gate layer, $i(t)$, decides which information is going to be updated. The tanh function creates a vector, $\tilde{C}(t)$, containing the new candidate values to be added to the state:

$$i(t) = \sigma\left(W_i \cdot \left[h(t-1), \mathbb{K}(t)\right] + b_i\right) \tag{5.15}$$

$$\tilde{C}(t) = \tanh\left(W_c \cdot \left[h(t-1), \mathbb{K}(t)\right] + b_c\right) \tag{5.16}$$

where W_i, b_i, W_c, and b_c denote the weights and bias of the sigmoid and tanh function, respectively. The memory gate produces the current memory $C(t)$, multiplying the old memory state, $Cs(t-1)$, by $fg(t)$, forgetting what was decided to be forgotten in the first step. Then, it is added by the multiplication of $i(t)$ with the new candidate values $\tilde{C}(t)$. This can be seen in the following equation:

$$C(t) = fg(t) \cdot C(t-1) + i(t) \cdot \tilde{C}(t) \tag{5.17}$$

The final step occurs in the output gate, $o(t)$, where the decision of the output is made. As in previous steps, a sigmoid layer decides which parts of the cell state are going to the output. Then, a tanh layer pushes the values from the cell state to be between −1 and 1, and multiplies it by the output of the sigmoid gate. This can be computed as follows:

$$o(t) = \sigma\left(W_o \cdot \left[h(t-1), \mathbb{K}(t)\right] + b_o\right) \tag{5.18}$$

$$h(t) = o(t) * \tanh\left(C(t)\right) \tag{5.19}$$

where $o(t)$ is the output gate activation and $h(t)$ is the neuron output at a certain instant t. W_o and b_o represent the weights and bias, respectively, within the output gate.

As already said before, LSTM has a chain structure just like RNN. However, instead of having a simple layer, each module has three gate layers containing sigmoid activation functions that constitute smooth curves between 0 and 1, making the module to remain differentiable. Apart from these gates, there is $\tilde{C}(t)$ that modifies the cell state. To calculate the candidate values, it uses a tanh function that with a zero–centred scale along with some operations will better distribute the gradients, allowing the network to remember for longer periods, i.e., retaining the information for longer periods without vanishing. If we consider the previous example, where the objective was to classify whether a player was attacking, defending, or counter-attacking, and take into account that the model can decide whether to keep the information that flows from cell to cell until it reaches the end of the network, it is more likely that the LSTM will correctly distinguish and classify if the player is, for example, attacking or counter-attacking, than the traditional RNN might be. To sum it up, while traditional RNN tussles to learn from long-term dependencies, LSTM's ability to forget, remember, and update the information pushes it one step ahead.

Non-Sequence vs Sequence Classification: The Golf Putting Use Case

Given the dynamic and complex nature of sports, it seems reasonable to calculate a set of 'static' features from time-dependent variables to simplify the analysis of the performance. In sports science, many denote these as process variables, which are related to the execution of the task (e.g., work and power of the leg muscles in football kicking), and product variables, which are related to the result of such task (e.g., accuracy and precision of the ball related to the goal). Selecting the most appropriate representative process and product variables is key in understanding the athletic performance, especially because the loss of information from their time-dependent counterpart is inevitable. For instance, Figure 5.1 depicts a practical example where process variables were considered, such as T_i, A_i with $i = \{1,2,3\}$, which represent the duration and the amplitude of the angular velocity of the leg during a penalty kick. These were calculated from the angular velocity of the thigh $w_{thigh}(t)$ and the angular velocity of the lower leg $w_{lower}(t)$ time series. Even though T_i, A_i with $i = \{1,2,3\}$ are process variables related to the penalty kick and enough for many studies around the football kick, they are not as informative as the time-dependent variables $w_{thigh}(t)$ and $w_{lower}(t)$ from which these were extracted from. Two penalty kicks may lead to the same duration and amplitude for each phase of the movement, while still presenting variations in the angular velocities of both thigh and lower leg. If this discrepancy between time-dependent variables and 'static' ones computed out of these are relevant or not is intrinsic to each situation, being an entirely different question and one to be addressed adopting yet another sports-related example that might be simpler to understand: the golf putting.

The golf putting is defined as a light golf stroke made on the green in an effort to place the ball into the hole (Pelz, 2000), representing about 43% of the strokes in a golf game (Alexander & Kern, 2005). The reasons why the golf putting has been chosen in this book to compare non-sequence and sequence classification methods are as follows:

1 It is a widely studied gesture: not only it is possible to easily contextualize the results obtained by the classifiers, but there are several datasets available to the community.
2 When compared to other gestures, it is rather easy to model: Pelz (2000) showed that the golf putting is a pendulum movement described by a simplistic, and yet efficient, mathematical model.

These two reasons, added to the fact that the authors of this book have contributed with several in-depth studies around the golf putting (Couceiro, Dias et al., 2013; Dias & Couceiro, 2015), make it as the right choice to demonstrate the differences between these two pattern recognition types. Other sports, such as football, will be addressed in the next section.

Similarly to Figure 5.1, a general overview of the adopted benchmark comparing non-sequence classification with sequence classification for the particular case of the golf putting is depicted in Figure 5.9. For the sake of simplicity, only the angular x-position of the putting (i.e., trajectory of the putter along the horizontal line) has been considered since it is the most representative process variable of the gesture (Couceiro, Dias et al., 2013). While this feeds the sequence data classifier directly, i.e., $\mathbb{K}(t) = \{x_{putt}\}$, just like before, a feature extraction routine has been adopted to extract meaningful variables that might not be time-dependent. As presented in Couceiro, Dias et al. (2013), the approach falls on the mathematical modelling, more specifically curve fitting, of the angular x-position of the putting with a sum of sinusoid waves. In order not to let the complexity of the problem grow inappropriately, a function composed

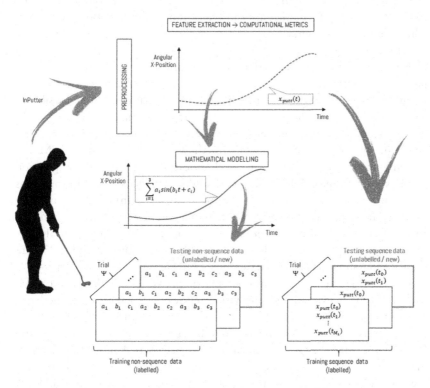

FIGURE 5.9 General classification approach applied to the golf putting.

by the sum of three sinusoids was used, $\sum_{i=1}^{3} a_i \sin(b_i t + c_i)$, thus leading to the set of 'static' features $Ж = \{a_i, b_i, c_i\} Ж = \{a_i, b_i, c_i\}$ with $i = \{1, 2, 3\}$.

Having the mathematical function defined as a sum of three sine waves, each of the three parameters of each wave needs to be estimated, resulting in a nine-dimensional estimation problem which attempts to minimize the mean squared estimation error for every experiment, in order to obtain an accurate mathematical function that describes the horizontal position of the golf club during putting execution (Couceiro, Dias et al., 2013). This is commonly known as curve fitting, although a more general, and adequate designation would be optimization. Briefly, optimization is the selection of the best element (with regard to some criteria) from some set of available alternatives. When applied, to fitting a given mathematical model to a real system, the optimization is the process of finding the optimal parameter of such model that has the best fit to a series of data points, possibly subject to constraints (Couceiro, Dias et al., 2013). This is out of the scope of this book, though more can be found in Dias and Couceiro (2015). Here, we hereby assume that this is an automatic process, where a set $Ж = \{a_i, b_i, c_i\}$ with $i = \{1, 2, 3\}$ is provided for each executed putting. Although it may sound like a hard assumption, some instruments available in the market are capable of providing this information with a high degree of efficiency, as is the case of the *InPutter* (Couceiro, Araújo, & Pereira, 2015).

Having said that, the objective of this example is simple: given a set of putting trials executed by different golf players, is it possible to extract a meaningful and unique playing signature, in such a way that it might be possible to automatically identify the player for new forthcoming trials?

To compare non-sequence and sequence classification applied to the same problem, two of the most renowned methods have been chosen: SVM and LSTM for non-sequence and sequence classification, respectively. A population of five volunteer male golfers who were adults, right-handed, and experts has been selected. Each performed 20 putting trials using InPutter at 4 m away from the hole. Put it differently, this example considers five classes – one for each player. The training dataset has been created with 75% of the trials randomly picked from the whole dataset (75 trials), whereas the remaining 25% are used as the testing dataset (25 trials).

Figure 5.10 compares the confusion matrix between both SVM and LSTM. The confusion matrix allows us to visualize the performance of the methods, wherein rows of the matrix represent the instances predicted by the methods and columns represent the targeted ones, being the latter provided as ground truth and only for the sake of evaluating the methods (Sokolova, Japkowicz, & Szpakowicz, 2006). The diagonal cells then correspond to observations that are correctly classified, i.e., putting trials that were never seen before and that

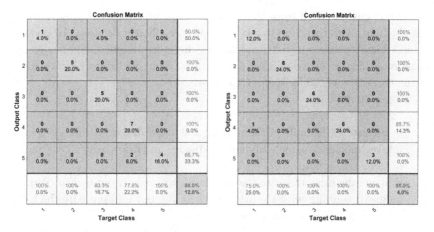

FIGURE 5.10   Confusion matrices: SVM (left), LSTM (right).

the methods were able to 'guess' which player executed them. However, the off-diagonal cells correspond to incorrectly classified observations, i.e., putting trials that were never seen before and that the methods were unable to 'guess' which player executed them. As one may observe, generally, the LSTM outperforms the SVM. Nevertheless, the SVM is still able to provide an overall accuracy of 88% (22 putting trials out of 25 correctly classified) against 96% of the LSTM (24 putting trials out of 25 correctly classified). However, the SVM was fed with only nine one-dimensional variables, against a time-dependent variable that can have more than 200 samples, if one considers the sampling frequency of 100 Hz provided by the InPutter device previously mentioned. Therefore, for a computational load considerably smaller when compared to the LSTM, the SVM is still able to provide promising results taking into account the dynamic nature of sports. It is, however, noteworthy that for time-dependent data, it highly relies on the computational metrics used to extract meaningful information.

A MatLab framework has been prepared for the purpose of running these and other experiments and evaluating non-sequence and sequence classifiers (Couceiro, 2020).

Human Action Recognition in Football

Unlike the golf putting described in the previous section, in football athletes can run on a straight line, side run, with quick changes of direction, with different velocities and rhythms (Dicharry, 2010). Such panoply of movements in only one action reveals how football can be challenging for action recognition. This area of studies became trendy with the promise of helping coaches, physiotherapists, and all team staff to understand how players behave during matches and, with that, lead to a faster and more efficient decision. To understand athlete's behaviour, independently of the sport practised, and as already mentioned, feature selection is key since some of them can be more informative than others as it was addressed in Chapter 4.

This section intends to:

1   Investigate the feasibility of combining and fusing data from different wearable technologies, namely Myontec's Mbody3 and Ingeniarius's TraXports, to recognize actions.
2   Evaluate the most adequate features for identifying actions such as (i) running, (ii) running with the ball, (iii) walking, (iv) walking with the ball, (v) passing, (vi) shooting, and (vii) jumping.
3   Compare the two sequence classification algorithms presented earlier in this chapter: LSTM and DBMM.

This study, fully described in Rodrigues et al. (2020), consisted of recording four futsal matches divided in a two-day tournament. Each of the four games had two 10-minute parts. Twenty-two injury-free males (22.2 ± 4.5 years, with max 39 years and min 19 years) have participated in this study. However, only one of them was equipped with a combination of the wearable technologies mentioned above. This allowed tracking both positional and physiological data. A video camera was also employed for a posterior ground-truth analysis, wherein recorded videos were synchronized with the wearables and, with that, it was possible to manually label the trials according to the action performed by the athlete.

Both LSTM and DBMM have been adopted and compared to investigate the feasibility of this solution. As supervised methods, and as described previously, both labelled training and testing datasets were needed to compare the result of both models with the expected result (ground-truth label). Table 5.1 presents the total number of trials for each action. This allows us to

TABLE 5.1 Number of trials for each different action/class

Actions	Number of trials
Running	183
Running with the ball	57
Walking	690
Walking with the ball	27
Passing	80
Shooting	15
Jumping	24

have representativeness of each action, or class, which justifies, to some extent, the performance of the methods in their identification.

As input data for the sequence classification methods, a total of nine time-dependent individual computational metrics, or features, were considered, including the athlete's (absolute) velocity, distance, and orientation towards the opponent goal, which were computed from kinematical data extracted from *TraXports*, and the normalized muscle activations values acquired from the athlete's lower limbs with Mbody3 (see the previous chapter). The feature selection was carried out before training and testing the model. Afterwards, the feature extraction was applied to the entire dataset, processing raw data into relevant time series to be used as input data.

In a first instance, the impact of each feature in the classification result was assessed by performing five tests containing the following combination for the classifier input $\mathbb{K}(t)$ for the LSTM:

Test 1 – EMG features:

$$\mathbb{K}(t) = \left\{ \begin{array}{l} EMG^1_i[t],\ EMG^2_i[t],\ EMG^3_i[t], \\ EMG^4_i[t],\ EMG^5_i[t],\ EMG^6_i[t] \end{array} \right\}$$

Test 2 – EMG and velocity:

$$\mathbb{K}(t) = \left\{ \begin{array}{l} EMG^1_i[t],\ EMG^2_i[t],\ EMG^3_i[t], \\ EMG^4_i[t],\ EMG^5_i[t],\ EMG^6_i[t],\ |v(t)| \end{array} \right\}$$

Test 3 – EMG and distance to the goal:

$$\mathbb{K}(t) = \left\{ \begin{array}{l} EMG^1_i[t],\ EMG^2_i[t],\ EMG^3_i[t], \\ EMG^4_i[t],\ EMG^5_i[t],\ EMG^6_i[t],\ d_g(t) \end{array} \right\}$$

Test 4 – EMG and orientation towards the goal:

$$\mathbb{K}(t) = \left\{ \begin{array}{l} EMG^1_i[t],\ EMG^2_i[t],\ EMG^3_i[t],\ EMG^4_i[t], \\ EMG^5_i[t],\ EMG^6_i[t],\ \theta_g(t) \end{array} \right\}$$

Test 5 – All features:

$$\mathbb{K}(t) = \left\{ \begin{array}{l} EMG^1_i[t],\ EMG^2_i[t],\ EMG^3_i[t],\ EMG^4_i[t], \\ EMG^5_i[t],\ EMG^6_i[t],\ |v(t)|,\ d_g(t),\ \theta_g(t) \end{array} \right\}$$

From the results obtained, it was possible to observe that the accuracy of LSTM increased from 59.6% to 60.13% by adding the velocity of the player to the EMG features. The same happened with the distance and orientation towards the opponent goal, having increased the model's accuracy by 1.07% and 0.21%, respectively. When all the features were used, the accuracy improvement of LSTM was 1.32% (see Figure 5.11). Refer to Sokolova et al. (2006) for more classification performance metrics and Rodrigues et al. (2020) for an in-depth discussion of these results.

Subsequently, the input dataset containing all the features was adopted to compare both LSTM and DBMM. To train and test the model more diversely, the process of splitting the data into training (70%) and test (30%) was repeated over 30 times, randomly. This also ensured that none of the training data was used for testing in order to avoid overfitting. A performance comparison between DBMM and LSTM is hereby shown in Figure 5.12, but in order to simplify it, one of the times was chosen where the model was trained and then tested. It shows that the DBMM performed better than the LSTM, reaching an overall accuracy of 88.5% against 66.1%, respectively.

This is an interesting use case since, in general, one would expect deep learning to outperform ensemble. This could be the case, however, if the dataset had a more consistent representation of each class, though, in this particular case, some classes were underrepresented when compared to others. For instance, the overall dataset had only 15 trials of the shooting action, though it had 690 trials for the action 'running with the ball'. Put it differently, it is known that LSTM, as a deep learning approach, requires a large representative dataset. However, while some of the actions were well represented in the dataset, others were not. This justifies the behaviour observed in the confusion matrix of the LSTM model (Figure 5.12), where the accuracy discrepancies of the different actions were substantial, making the learning

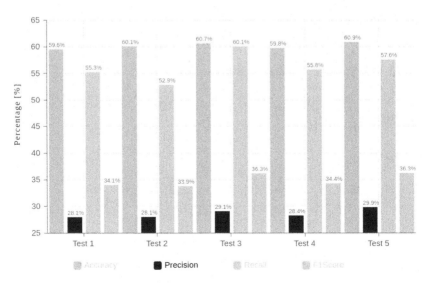

FIGURE 5.11 Evaluation metrics per test (adapted from Rodrigues et al. (2020)).

Confusion Matrix

Output Class	Running	Running w/ ball	Passing	Walking	Walking w/ ball	Shoting	Jumping	
Running	45 / 14.0%	1 / 0.3%	2 / 0.6%	7 / 2.2%	0 / 0.0%	0 / 0.0%	0 / 0.0%	81.1% / 18.9%
Running w/ ball	1 / 0.3%	13 / 4.0%	1 / 0.3%	2 / 0.6%	0 / 0.0%	0 / 0.0%	0 / 0.0%	75.7% / 24.3%
Passing	1 / 0.3%	0 / 0.0%	16 / 5.0%	2 / 0.6%	0 / 0.0%	0 / 0.0%	0 / 0.0%	84.1% / 15.9%
Walking	8 / 2.5%	3 / 0.9%	5 / 1.6%	195 / 60.6%	1 / 0.3%	1 / 0.3%	1 / 0.3%	91.1% / 8.9%
Walking w/ ball	0 / 0.0%	0 / 0.0%	0 / 0.0%	1 / 0.3%	7 / 2.2%	0 / 0.0%	0 / 0.0%	81.5% / 18.5%
Shoting	0 / 0.0%	0 / 0.0%	0 / 0.0%	0 / 0.0%	0 / 0.0%	3 / 0.9%	0 / 0.0%	81.7% / 13.8%
Jumping	0 / 0.0%	0 / 0.0%	0 / 0.0%	0 / 0.0%	0 / 0.0%	0 / 0.0%	6 / 1.9%	87.6% / 12.4%
	81.2% / 18.8%	76.5% / 23.5%	66.6% / 33.4%	94.0% / 6.0%	85.8% / 14.2%	68.0% / 32.0%	79.9% / 20.1%	88.5% / 11.5%

Target Class

Confusion Matrix

Output Class	Running	Running w/ ball	Passing	Walking	Walking w/ ball	Shoting	Jumping	
Running	7 / 2.2%	4 / 1.2%	2 / 0.6%	13 / 4.0%	0 / 0.0%	0 / 0.0%	0 / 0.0%	26.9% / 73.1%
Running w/ ball	2 / 0.6%	2 / 0.6%	3 / 0.9%	2 / 0.6%	1 / 0.3%	1 / 0.3%	0 / 0.0%	18.2% / 81.8%
Passing	1 / 0.3%	0 / 0.0%	14 / 4.3%	3 / 0.9%	2 / 0.6%	1 / 0.3%	2 / 0.6%	60.9% / 39.1%
Walking	43 / 13.4%	10 / 3.1%	0 / 0%	187 / 58.1%	5 / 1.6%	1 / 0.3%	2 / 0.6%	75.4% / 24.6%
Walking w/ ball	0 / 0.0%	0 / 0.0%	0 / 0.0%	1 / 0.3%	0 / 0.0%	0 / 0.0%	0 / 0.0%	0.0% / 100%
Shoting	2 / 0.6%	1 / 0.3%	3 / 0.9%	1 / 0.3%	0 / 0.0%	0 / 0.0%	0 / 0.0%	0.0% / 100%
Jumping	0 / 0.0%	0 / 0.0%	2 / 0.6%	0 / 0.0%	0 / 0.0%	1 / 0.3%	3 / 0.9%	50.0% / 50.0%
	12.7% / 87.3%	11.8% / 88.2%	58.3% / 41.7%	90.3% / 9.7%	0.0% / 100%	0.0% / 100%	42.9% / 57.1%	66.1% / 33.9%

Target Class

FIGURE 5.12   Confusion matrices: (top) DBMM, (bottom) LSTM.

process of the algorithm and its consequent decision very much influenced by the class/action containing a larger amount of data, being this the main reason why the LSTM network presented an inferior performance compared to the DBMM.

Conclusion

Two types of AI approaches for pattern recognition in sports were introduced: non-sequence and sequence classification. Non-sequence classification deals with 'static' data, where each sample is described by a set of features, each having a fixed dimension. A sequence classification approach is characterized by its variable-sized features, where each sample can be represented by one or more features with changing values over time. Most of the time, non-sequence classification problems can be characterized by independent situations. In a sports context, it can be the number of times a movement is performed. Nevertheless, certain dynamic movements can still be modelled, or process variables extracted out of those and fed to non-sequence classifiers. Regarding sequence classification problems, it can be characterized by evolving situations, i.e., the movement that was performed during a certain time interval.

As expected, the more powerful the machine learning algorithm, the more complex the problem that they can deal with; deep learning methods are known for their outstanding performance. However, this benefit comes at the cost of requiring more training data; thus, larger computational resources are required. Deep learning approaches are known for their high GPU requirements, being the most resource-intensive task in the whole pattern recognition cycle. Moreover, if the data is not well represented, deep learning methods may even perform worse than other approaches since highly imbalanced datasets pose added difficulty, leading the methods to exhibit a bias towards the majority class, and, in extreme cases, even ignore the minority class altogether.

6

FROM CLASSIFICATION TO PREDICTION

Introduction

As Chapter 5 addressed, classification aims to identify an object's class through a classification model trained with significant information on a data sample. The model built, based on a certain dataset, is then used to classify values of untested data. Prediction, however, focuses on forecasting, for example, an unseen variable value. The latter is often addressed when the input data is time-related, i.e., when the data is a sequence of observations over time. The predictive model observes each element of the sequence and tries to predict its value according to the previous observations.

Analysing time-related events opens plenty of possibilities for companies or sports teams as it can help them to forecast events, such as winning or losing a game, or predict the customer's behaviour. In football, predicting the outcome of a match can be challenging since it relies on many factors (Owramipur, Eskandarian, & Mozneb, 2013). From a statistical point of view, being able to predict whether a team is going to score or even how many goals are going to be scored is an important feature, especially for the betting market (Spann & Skiera, 2009). For bettors, the outcome of a match is decided not only by the position of the team in the league, but also by other underlying performance indicators, or features, that may say more about that team and its players. Thus, and according to the literature, predictions need to make use of the past information, i.e., information known from past actions, and combine it with other factors, such as home advantage, teamwork, weather, number of injuries, and individual or collective performance, among others (Razali, Mustapha, Yatim, & Ab Aziz, 2017). This represents a huge amount of real-time data that can be used and non-linearly combined to predict whatever can happen next. However, such huge amount of data leads, again, to the 'Big Data' problem

(Chapter 1), which is far too complex for humans to handle, making the choice of the right computational metrics and artificial intelligence methods crucial (Sillanpää & Heino, 2013). Another critical aspect, namely related to football, is that, in most occasions, these approaches require a large number of different situations to occur over time. For instance, to predict whether a team will either win or lose a given match against another team may require a large amount of data from both teams, preferably even from both teams playing together. This is particularly difficult since team players, coaches, and playing strategies change constantly over different seasons. Moreover, even during a large league, such as the Premier League, each team plays (only) 38 matches, being still considered as a rather small sample size, thus making it difficult to strip out of the randomness of a football game from the equation.

According to Gama, Dias, Passos, Couceiro, and Davids (2020), artificial intelligence methods have the potential to facilitate the understanding of football, namely regarding its inherent performance dynamics, and, with that, increase their practical applicability and predictability. Being able to predict the outcome of a game, as well as predicting possible injuries within a match, is one of the main goals of this type of research, regardless of how unpredictable a football match can be (Couceiro et al., 2016; Gama et al., 2020). For instance, injuries can be the result of contact and non-contact events. Contact-based injuries are related to external factors, such as physical collisions and tackles. Injuries caused by non-contact events are, for example, injuries occurring during running, making those easier to be predicted than the former. Besides predicting injuries, knowing how long the player will need to get back from the injury is a factor of interest not only for the medical team but also for the coach, allowing the latter to better organize the team (Kampakis, 2013). To investigate the possibility of predicting injuries, many computational methods have been studied, including machine learning approaches, agent-based and system dynamics, and neural network's techniques (Fonseca et al., 2020; Gama et al., 2020).

There are plenty of factors, such as physiological, biomechanical, social, psychological, and environmental variables, that, when properly combined, can provide the necessary cues to forecast different football phenomena (Fonseca et al., 2020). For instance, one factor that has been studied over the last years is the home advantage (Courneya & Carron, 1992). According to Leite (2017), the home advantage intrinsically contemplates other related factors that can greatly influence the performance of the teams in the field, such as the crowd, the familiarity with the field, and the effect of the displacement travels of visitor's teams. Furthermore, there is a psychological aspect that reinforces the idea that home teams believe on the advantage of playing at home, which gives them more confidence and, therefore, they naturally play at their best. Confidence, however, is yet another factor that considerably influences the team's performance; according to Goddard and Asimakopoulos (2004), the participation in external cups, as well as championships and promotions, are determinants in a football outcome. Not as significant as confidence, or with less emphasis on the literature, other psychological factors, such as high anxiety, tension, fatigue, and demotivation, can also have a negative impact on players, affecting their performance (Campo et al., 2019). Fatigue, for instance, is considered as an important factor that can influence the football player's skills, affecting both technique and tactic performance (Stone & Oliver, 2009). From a psychological point of view, the burnout effect can lead to emotional and physical exhaustion, a reduced sense of accomplishment, and an uncaring and cynical attitude towards sport participation (Raedeke & Smith, 2001).

Again, as before, prediction can be achieved by adopting sequential or non-sequential methods. However, instead of classifying a class with the respective label, as done in classification, the objective is to predict what may happen next considering what has happened before. The next section explores the convergence analysis of the sequence classification methods DBMM and LSTM, addressed in the previous chapter, to assess whether a fast prediction may be seen as a short-term prediction. Later in this section, we relate seemingly farfetched variables, using the distribution of passes to predict the number of goal attempts and goals scored (Gama et al., 2020).

Convergence Analysis

Convergence analysis is one key factor to understand the performance of artificial intelligence models as it reflects the algorithm's ability to adapt to a changing dynamic system (Yi, 2013). It can tell how fast the models converge to the targeted solution or even if they converge at all, thus showing its reliability. Studying the convergence of a system is an important part to assess its feasibility, so as to make sure whether it is a proper model to work with real-time data. It is important to know not only whether the model is converging properly, but also how fast it is able to predict the outcome. In sports, more specifically football, the convergence time of both DBMM and LSTM algorithms has been studied within the context of the work presented in the previous chapter (Section 'Human Action Recognition in Football') (Rodrigues et al., 2020), hereby described to illustrate its importance and whether these methods may be adopted for short-term predictions.

Within the context of classification, the convergence is described as the time interval that each algorithm takes from receiving data from a certain class to the moment in which the algorithm classifies it correctly, thus answering the question: *How long does it take for the model to correctly identify the true class of a certain input?* As explained in the previous chapter, both DBMM and LSTM models have been trained with a dataset of actions observed during a few matches. However, after having the model trained, instead of classifying each trial as a whole, the models have been fed each time step at a time with the intent to study their convergence and assess how long it takes them to identify the action performed by the athlete. The top images in Figures 6.1 and 6.2 depict the targeted class (action executed) overlaid by the predicted class (action predicted by the model) for DBMM and LSTM, respectively. Likewise, the bottom images in Figures 6.1 and 6.2 depict the targeted class (action executed) overlaid by the predicted probability of being from a given class (probability of a given action predicted by the model) for DBMM and LSTM, respectively.

Figure 6.2 shows that the LSTM model is unable to properly converge towards a given class, i.e., it is unable to reliable predict the right action. From the beginning, the LSTM seems to assume all input sequences as the walking action (class 4). As explained in Chapter 5, this misbehaviour is related to the fact that deep learning methods need to be fed by a large amount of

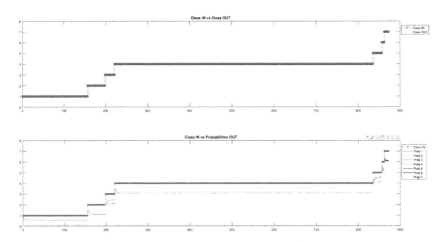

FIGURE 6.1 Convergence analysis of DBMM.

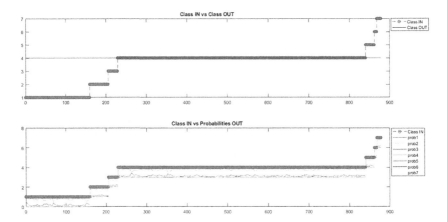

FIGURE 6.2 Convergence analysis of LSTM.

TABLE 6.1 Rise time of each different action/class

Classes	1	2	3	4	5	6	7
Time (s)	0	2.960	2.760	1.320	3.360	3.240	1.920

training data for each class, which was not the case. Besides the dataset source not being representative enough, the number of samples between classes was greatly unbalanced, favouring the walking action by far and, therefore, leading to the results herein presented. The convergence of the DBMM was considerably more consistent than the LSTM. One can observe in Figure 6.1 that the probability transition between classes allows us to easily assess the rise time (see Table 6.1) of each class, i.e., the time that the DBMM took from receiving the data until it was correctly classified (Table 6.1).

As is possible to observe, DBMM converges differently depending on the action it is trying to predict. Nonetheless, class 1, or running, was undoubtedly the action the model was able to predict faster, taking less than 1 s to identify it. On the other extreme, however, DBMM took more than 3 s to adequately identify whether the player was passing or shooting, bearing in mind that these were also the actions where the DBMM failed the most in recognizing them (see the previous chapter).

This information enlightens the importance of a convergence time analysis, especially for prediction problems, as it can tell us how long the model will take until forecasting an event, with a good degree of certainty. In other words, the faster the model is detecting, for example, an event, an incident, or a failure, the shorter the response time will be, and more room for decisions is left to the technical team and coaches. The current use case, however, also shows how limiting these approaches can be to identify an ongoing event by using individual computational metrics computed directly out of kinematical and psychological data. The next section goes beyond these limitations by exploring prediction methods on group metrics.

Predicting the Number of Goal Attempts and Goals Scored

As stated before, sport prediction, whether it is the outcome of a football match or the detections of a possible injury, can provide important information about the individual and the group performance of athletes. Yet, finding the right representative patterns, or features, is one of the most important tasks for this matter. One expects such features to represent the dynamics of sports, assessing differences between the team and the individual behaviour of athletes and, ultimately, to forecast what can possibly happen next.

The recently published work of Gama et al. (2020) showed the relationship between the homogeneity of passes between players from the same team and the number of goal attempts and goals scored. The homogeneity of passes is there described as a feature that intends to represent a performance measure, defined as a balanced distribution of passes made and received during a match. However, this is not as trivial as it sounds. This performance measure can be influenced by the structure of the team, being affected by many factors, such as the position of the team players. In Gama et al. (2020), the authors build a non-linear relationship with the number of passes and the team's ability to move within the field. The authors' rationale is that the more dynamic the players are, the larger the possibility of creating passing lines, thus dismantling the opposite team defence strategy and, with that, increasing the possibility of scoring.

In a nutshell, Gama et al. (2020) considered a dataset of ten official football matches of ten Portuguese professional football teams from the Portuguese Premier League from the 2010/2011 season. From the dataset, the authors analysed 2,578 collective offensive actions, 6,100 successful passes and crosses between the offensive players, 165 shots on goal and 15 goals. Interactions between teammates, therein represented by passes, have been quantified by applying Shannon's entropy directly to the 14 × 14 (11 titular and 3 substitutes) adjacency matrix of passes (see Chapter 4 for an explanation on how to generate the adjacency matrix based on inter-player interactions). The entropy itself is a direct measure of the amount of information within a variable, which, in this case, would represent the discrepancy of passes made between pairs of players, i.e., the variability of the distribution of passes. Put it differently, the higher the entropy values, the higher the variability of the number of passes and vice versa.

Having the time sequence analysis in mind, the adjacency matrix, and related entropy, was calculated over a 5-minute sliding window, wherein the latter was then fed to a time-delay neural network. The neural network was trained based on two different target outputs: the number of goal attempts and goals scored. A delay time of 1 minute was chosen, meaning that the method would be expect to predict the number of goal attempts and goals scored 1 minute before happening. For the sake of evaluating the proposed methodology, the last match (tenth match) was not used during the training phase, being only considered for the validation phase. Pearson's linear correlation was applied to quantify the accuracy of the machine learning method, i.e., to assess how accurate were the output predictions comparing to the ground truth.

Figure 6.3 depicts the behaviour of the predictive model to predict goal attempts using the mean entropy values of passing distribution as the input time series.

The bottom image in Figure 6.3 represents the sliding window data of goal attempts observed in the tenth match which was not used for training. The black dashed line represents the prediction of goal attempts whereas the filled grey line outlines the actual number of goal attempts. As one can see, the model considered in this work was able to identify a pattern between variables, goal

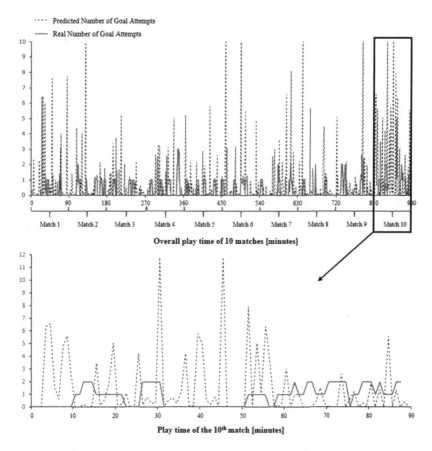

FIGURE 6.3 Predicted number of goal attempts using the mean entropy values of passing distribution (Gama et al., 2020).

attempts, and the entropy of passing distribution, in such a way that it could predict the possibility of occurring a goal attempt over a 1-minute timeframe. Having a closer look at the zoomed section, one can notice that the prediction occurs before the real events happened, which shows its ability to anticipate occurrences within a match. Pearson's linear correlation coefficients for every match in the dataset showed a positive linear relationship between the prediction of goal attempts while using the entropy and the real goal attempts.

Likewise, the same procedure has been adopted for goals scored. However, due to the small number of goals, which leads to a lack of representativeness of this particular product variable, the method was unable to perform as well as with goal attempts. Yet, the results of this case study still exhibited a relationship between the homogeneity of passing distribution and the goal attempts (Figure 6.4).

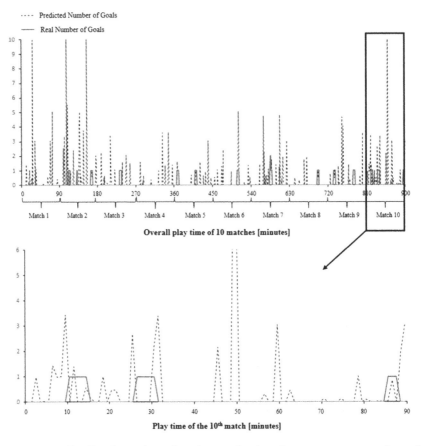

FIGURE 6.4 Predicted number of goals scored using the mean entropy values of passing distribution (Gama et al., 2020).

Conclusion

This chapter introduced the concept of prediction in sports, namely football, extending the classification problem for on-the-fly performance analysis. The key motivation behind the development of predictive models in sports falls on the need to predict certain outcomes beforehand, be it for performance assessment or for injury prevention, which can then support coaches' decision-making.

Two different approaches were described as use cases: (i) predict actions performed by a player during matches based on individual metrics; (ii) predict the number of goal attempts and goals scored during matches based on group metrics. The results show that there is a gap between classification and prediction since many factors contribute to the unpredictability inherent to sports. Like classification, however, prediction also relies on the adoption of adequate artificial intelligence model and representative features.

7

TECHNOLOGY, ARTIFICIAL INTELLIGENCE, AND THE FUTURE OF SPORT AND PHYSICAL ACTIVITY

Introduction

This chapter concludes the book by summarizing the main contributions.

In recent years, understanding of performance in sport, as well as the capacity to track data of people engaged in recreational-level physical activity and exercise, has rapidly developed (Couceiro et al., 2016). In co-authoring this book, we sought to understand how AI can be used to enhance and enrich participation in sport and physical activity from the perspectives of high performance and lifelong recreational engagement. The chapters of this book examined different aspects of artificial intelligence, which require digital technologies to provide support for tasks – such as education, coaching, teaching, and supporting learning and performance in sport and physical activities – that have traditionally challenged humans. The book indicates how the current focus of attention in AI research has been to create and develop hardware and software systems that can record, classify, analyse, and interpret large amounts of data. In sport, there has been a considerable amount of effort undertaken for providing a wide range of ever-improving technological solutions designed to extract data about key aspects of performance during training and competition, including kinematics of movement, collective system behaviours, and physiological data on outputs of different sub-systems.

An important take-home message from the book is that the AI system implementation and exploitation stages require teams of specialists working in a transdisciplinary organization to act on data, for the purposes of continuously enhancing athlete learning, development, and performance preparation from augmented information provided from AI systems (Rothwell, Davids, Stone, Araújo, & Shuttleworth, 2020). The implementation of new digital tools for recording, analysing, and tracking of information on individual's performance, progression, and health has enhanced the use of artificial intelligence systems to augment the (re)design of selection, training, and practice activities, supporting an individualization of such processes as never before. Summarizing the technical engineering advances in sport, Couceiro et al. (2016) noted how such intelligence systems provided data and feedback to regulate athlete behaviours by enhancing: (i) development of innovative technological solutions to estimate the changing location of wearable mobile devices in a performance setting, supporting individual tracking with multi-lateration techniques and wireless propagation measures; (ii) design of multi-sensor fusion algorithms to provide real-time and fault-tolerant information about an individual's organizational state (i.e., position and orientation), integrating wireless propagation measures with data coming from attached inertial measurement units; (iii) integration of physiological sensors during exercise and training (e.g., heart rate monitors) within wearable devices for non-invasive remote bio-signal monitoring of the active individual's performance state and design of data mining procedures to improve data reliability from the sensing units; and (iv) with regard to sport performance, mathematical formulations of software systems for online performance analysis and predictions based on player actions, locations, and physiological data monitored over time.

In this chapter, we overview the key 'take-home' messages that may be highlighted from reading this text. At one level of analysis, an important message is to warn against *technological determinism*: considering new technological advances as an immutable over-arching force that imposes irresistible and unavoidable changes on the functional behaviours of individuals, organizations, communities, and societies. Despite the enormous amounts of funding devoted to finding technological solutions to planning and predicting outcomes of competitive events, sports still have a significant amount of uncertainty. This sentiment is captured by Brazil's assistant national coach, Sylvinho, discussing how the margins between winning and losing can be wafer-thin (https://www.theguardian.com/football/2020/aug/03/sylvinho-winning-a-treble-with-barcelona-was-spectacular-arsenal-wenger-guardiola-manager). Here, he discussed how some of the greatest coaches in association football including Pep Guardiola, Tite national coach of Brazil, and Roberto Mancini could never guarantee winning competitions:

> Guardiola used to always say: 'Lads, we're going to do everything, everything, everything, everything. But I don't know if we'll win, I can't guarantee that.' Tite's the same: he studies all… day … long. Locked away, studying. Mancini too, moving with the game. I see Diego Simeone, a great coach, lose two European Cup finals. Sometimes, the difference between winning or not is tiny. We won a treble getting there via Stamford Bridge with the last kick. Bloody hell. Pffff. How do you explain that?

Furthermore, it is important to recognize that the rapid proliferation of digital technologies in physical education, sport, and physical activity also risks an over-reliance on its use. For more effective implementation of technology, it needs to be integrated into a methodology for enhancing performance and enriching the development of athletes and teams (Stone, Strafford, North, Toner, & Davids, 2018).

Artificial Intelligence Needs a Powerful Conceptualization of Performance, Learning, and Development in Sport and Physical Activity

The unpredictability of competitive sport comes about because there are just too many variables, which could potentially impact on performance, rendering AI in need of support to enhance its use in guiding performance preparation and athlete development. In short, technology can produce copious amounts of data, which can be used to support performance of athletes and teams. But its implementation needs a comprehensive theoretical framework to interpret the statistical values and make the most of the patterns and structures in the information available in large sets of data (Stone et al., 2018).

How Ecological Dynamics Can Help Make Sense of Big Data from AI Systems

Indeed, the chapters of this book suggest how massive technological changes felt over the past few years have led to a new issue: captured in the term *big data*. A prevailing assumption has been that developing methods to collect data will complement analytic methods to improve sport performance in significant ways, such as tuning training plans or determining performance patterns of competitors. An important challenge for sport scientists and practitioners is to develop a selective understanding of which data matter and how to interpret them from the massive banks of available information, leading to coherent use in supporting training, performance preparation, and talent development systems. This is an important issue to understand since implementation of AI systems and technologies during training, exercise, and performance has become standard leading to the availability of huge amounts of information for athletes, sport practitioners, and coaches. In fact, collecting and accessing so much data from various types of system analyses is a real opportunity for scientists and practitioners because they can get new performance information that was not available in the past. But it's also a risk having too much data, which requires implementation of data or dimension reduction by sport scientists, using techniques from AI (e.g., machine and deep learning). In the meantime, an underlying risk of data reduction and data modelling is to lose the meaning of the context behind the large datasets for practitioners. This is because, when fuzzing data, reducing dimension, and modelling parameters, the outcome can be hugely challenging and complex to understand and interpret for coaches and sport practitioners, making the transfer from the dataset to intervention design not straightforward. The challenges posed by AI implementation in sport and physical activity are captured by the following questions: what do these datasets mean for performance, learning, and development of individual athletes? How can these sources of information be used to help individuals improve performance over time? What sort of theoretical conceptualization of athlete and team performance and development can help us to make sense of the data and use the information to benefit individuals in sport at all levels of performance and expertise?

Practitioners' work needs to be data-informed, not data-driven. This book advances the argument that *data-informed* decision-making is needed to engage learners, trainers, and performers, instead of *data-driven* approaches, requiring a comprehensive theoretical framework to critically interpret the information from the large and complex datasets for enriching athlete behaviours before, during, and after training and in competition. Indeed, sensors always provide data to scientists and practitioners, even when those data may be poorly collected, poorly reflecting the core of practice and perhaps collected during a decontextualized or non-representative training protocol, compounding the weakness of data-driven approaches.

A key contention is that experiences of individuals participating in sport, physical activity, and exercise, from a recreational to an elite level, can be enriched or demeaned by the implementation of new technologies. This issue was originally examined in the study of implementing advanced digital technologies into manufacturing production (Jackson & Wall, 1991). Research on the implementation of advanced manufacturing technologies into existing process manufacturing settings revealed that a theoretical framework for the implementation of work design was needed to ensure maintenance of operator performance and well-being. Evidence suggested the importance of theoretical understanding of human performance behaviours (including motivation, skill expression, and problem-solving) in allowing operators to use their skills appropriately in the production process, rather than de-skilling them in favour of adopting what was called a 'technology as superstar' mentality in work organization. The findings also indicated the potential of a collaborative relationship between engineers, technical specialists, and operator skills trainers in enriching the work environment (Davids & Wall, 1990). In sport, these ideas have important implications for continuous collaborations between specialist support staff, including coaches, trainers, sport scientists, data scientists, engineers, and performance analysts, in a Department of Methodology (Rothwell et al., 2020) for designing learning and training environments for individuals in sport and physical activity programmes at different expertise levels, which we discuss later in this chapter.

What these findings suggest is that the challenge of developing active individuals and athletes, and improving sport performance or levels of participation, is closely related to the use of technology in designing environments that continuously enrich the engagement of individual athletes in their participation activities. Principles of this engagement process are the same for a world champion athlete preparing to compete or a child learning to move in a PE class, with the key differences residing within the nature of the specifying information and affordances present within each individual's performance landscape.

An Ecological Dynamics Conceptualization of Human Behaviour: Implications for Use of AI Systems in Sport

In Chapter 1, we discussed how an ecological dynamics framework for sport scientists, educators, and practitioners can support the interpretation of large datasets collected from athlete behaviours in practice and performance, which can help coaches and trainers design better practice tasks and sustain evidence-based interpretations of athlete performance in sport. The aim of enriching participatory experiences is fundamentally an embedded process of using technological support to continuously promote individual interactions with sport, exercise, and physical activity environments (Reed, 1993; Renshaw et al., 2019; Stone et al., 2018; Woods, McKeown, Shuttleworth, Davids, & Robertson, 2019). The ontology of ecological realism underpins ecological dynamics as an important framework for understanding learning, practice, education, and development, from a perspective that emphasizes search exploration, discovery, re-organization, stabilization, and exploitation of knowledge of a performance environment for regulating actions. New technologies can support provision of real-time or short-term feedback and monitoring, which could help the regulation of actions, favouring behavioural adaptability in performance. For instance, use of miniaturized inertial measurement units allows continuous data collection during ecological contexts of performance that enables sport practitioners to detect perturbations (performance and/or behavioural destabilizations) developing flexibility and adaptive behaviours in athletes (for an example, see Guignard et al., 2017b).

Technology Implementation Should Drive Knowledge of the Environment in Athletes

Chapter 1 is fundamentally important to understanding key concepts of psychological theories of human behaviour that underpin implementation of AI technologies for use in sport, physical activity, and exercise contexts. That chapter outlined the role of these technologies in the evolution and development of the ability to use affordances of the environment that are fundamental to successful performance in the human econiche. According to James Gibson, perception is a fundamental type of cognition, and aligned with these ideas, Turvey and Carello (1981) pointed out that cognition, from the ontological perspective of ecological realism, may be considered as the coordination of an individual's intentional interactions with the affordances of a performance environment. Reed (1993) elegantly explained how psychological processes underpinning cognition could support *knowledge of* an environment, describing how it is provided by perception allowing an organism (sport performer) to be aware of events, objects, and significant others that exist (attention, perception), have existed (memories), may come to exist (anticipation), and ought to exist (prediction) during interactions. Reed's (1993) insights can be taken to imply that actions, perception, and cognition of athletes during performance and practice are 'knowledge-yielding processes' (p. 47). In the many chapters of this book, we have outlined how AI systems can be implemented to provide augmented information in support of the knowledge-based functioning of athletes during their interactions with practice and performance environments.

Knowledge about Sport Performance and Practice: The Role of AI

At a most basic level, artificial intelligence provides information to help people 'know what to do' in specific environments, forming their intentions and goals, as the basis of 'cognition' in sport behaviours (Araújo, Hristovski, et al., 2019). James Gibson (1979), the founder of the ecological approach, argued that cognition is ecological. This is because an environment is to be perceived, acted upon, cognised, and shared between people collaborating on specific intentions, which may be captured in performance goals. An ecological conceptualization of cognition is active, shared, and outward looking, forming the basis of continuous interactions with the environment. In Chapter 1 we noted that perception is a cognitive function of the most basic kind because it yields knowledge of *affordances* (opportunities for action) of the performance environment.

In this viewpoint, acquiring detailed and substantial *knowledge about* a performance environment is an excellent foundation upon which to use AI to build athlete performance and development. In an ecological dynamics rationale of cognition, the environment is to be perceived, acted upon, and known by an athlete seeking to interact with its key task constraints such as rules, space, other performers, equipment, surfaces, and conditions. Here we proposed how the role of AI is to support and enrich the cognition of the environment during performance and practice, providing data to supplement coach and athlete interactions. Artificial intelligence provided by new technologies is best implemented for use in practice and performance environments that are to be perceived, acted upon, and known by athletes and teams seeking to interact with key performance constraints. The intended direction for using skills and knowledge is the basis of any athlete's perception and use of affordances that surround him/her. An important role of AI in sport contexts is through supporting cognitions of an individual performer, regardless of skill level and expertise. Cognition is considered to frame the way that 'any and all psychological processes' (Reed, 1993, p. 46) may function in providing *knowledge of* the environment, especially with respect to being situated for interacting with a performance context.

These ideas from Reed (1993) suggest how affordances and an individual's intentionality are the key to understanding how cognition may be used for understanding an environment. People's specific intentions are so important for using affordances and in collective groups these intentions can be shared or jointly perceived. Intentions help select a sub-group of available affordances, from the multitude available, to be used to underpin selected actions. Attention and actions can support this selections process. Intentionality of direction for using skills and *knowledge of* the environment is the basis of any individual's use of affordances that surround him/her. Of course, this selection of affordances to achieve specific intentions does not occur in a vacuum. For example, socio-cultural constraints influence this continuous selection of affordances, constituting a form of life (Rothwell et al., 2020). Reed (1993, p. 49) proposed: 'As the environment to be acted upon changes, the developing person him or herself changes, reorganizing his or her action systems'. The constraints which shape these interactions include not only biophysical surrounds but also socio-cultural and historical constraints constituting a form of life continually shaped by family, peer group, organizations, trends, changing technologies, societies and communities, and educational experiences. Reed (1993) noted that it is the perception and use of affordances that can become culturally biased, but not the affordances themselves.

In contrast, James Gibson (1979) argued that *knowledge about* the environment is more abstract, symbolic, and cultural, relating to numerical, linguistic, gestural communication which can help in re-organizing and securing knowledge gained via perception which can be used in more abstract form. Human understanding involves different combinations of several modes of cognition. Whereas coaches, trainers, and sport science support staff exist in a professional organization of data from practice and performance formed by *knowledge about* things like actions, outcomes, performance data, physiological effects on the sub-systems of the body, in contrast athletes inhabit performance environment preferencing *knowledge of* the environment for interactions. In this sense, the information provided by AI systems needs to be translated by sport practitioners in order for the data to be used by athletes during practice and performance, since both groups have different knowledge sources, and therefore perspectives, for knowing what to do. This nexus of knowledge about AI and knowledge of performance constitutes an innovative crux point in this book.

What Are the Key Messages from the Chapters of This Book?

The discussion of performance analysis stressed the importance of performance analysis in sports under three different perspectives: (i) the researcher, (ii) the coach and technical teams, and (iii) the athlete. It describes the relevance of recording and measuring athlete performance and behaviours during competition, training, practice, recovery, and rest. The chapters have provided a discussion around one of the most recent and relevant concerns in sports: how to deal with *big data*. This discussion will provide a summary of recent approaches adopted to improve the interpretation of large and complex volumes of data in order to avoid falling back into the mere *datafication* of information in exercise, physical activity, and sports, thus leading away from traditional methods for quantifying sport performances to a pattern-driven quantification that was further described in later chapters.

In *Chapter 2* we discussed recent data analytics perspectives settled on the detection of spatiotemporal, patterned structures of data in sport performance, based on the assumption that complex streams of human behaviour, in individual or collective performance contexts, have a sequential structure. That chapter described the limitations of traditional methods for quantifying sport performance in their capacity to capture the complex patterns that emerge in sport performance over time, and under specific constraints. It outlined novel approaches that have been adopted for the analysis of spatiotemporal patterns of interactions between competitors and teammates in sports, regardless of whether those patterns emerged from individual perceptual-motor systems, or from time-based events, and other contexts. The chapter highlighted how the AI research community has begun to pay attention to the context of sport performance as an important arena for analysing statistical patterns in large datasets for the purposes of improving performance preparation and developing athletes. The major focus has been on developing specialized machine learning algorithms and analytical procedures for selecting individuals and designing specific training programmes to fulfil athlete and team potential.

Later chapters elucidated how analysis of performance of sports teams and athletes requires dynamic pattern analysis of large datasets. It highlighted recent data analysis perspectives, focused on the detection of spatiotemporal structures of data in sports, under the assumption that complex streams of human behaviour, be it individual or collective, have a sequential structure. It described the limitations of traditional methods for quantifying sport performance in their capacity to describe the complex patterns emerging in sports over time. It outlined novel approaches that have been adopted for the analysis of spatiotemporal patterns of interactions in sports, exemplified by movement patterns, time-based events, and interactions between individuals in sub-groups. For instance, some great advantages of gathering a massive bank of data, such as long time series of measures during training, acquired with various types of sensors (e.g., GPS, IMU, heart rate sensor), include the following:

i Tracking the performance and/or the behavioural dynamics instead of going with static or discrete event analyses. Thus, AI techniques enable sport practitioners to scan the whole action repertoire of an athlete/team, non-linearity and non-proportionality phenomena in the dynamics (e.g., bifurcation, critical fluctuations, hysteresis, multi-stability, indicators of complexity, entropy) (Komar, Seifert, & Thouvarecq, 2015; Seifert, Button, & Davids, 2013). Therefore, one real 'value added' of AI is to detect, quantify, and/or qualify phenomena that cannot be perceived and assessed through human observation, but that exist and could reveal important aspects of expertise, learning, adaptive behaviours, well-being, or injury risks.

ii Assessing and understanding intra- and inter-individual sources of variability. Indeed, movement and coordination variability has traditionally been considered as a type of system 'noise' characterized by a deviation from an 'expert' technique or template. Recent advanced analyses in AI, using unsupervised machine learning techniques (i.e., without any *a priori* outputs to avoid human bias), have highlighted the functional role of variability in sport performance (Seifert & Davids, 2012). For instance, cluster analysis methodologies illustrate how intra- and inter-individual variability of movement pattern coordination could be functional as it corresponds to individual adaptations when interacting with a set of constraints (Rein, Button, Davids, & Summers, 2010; for an example in swimming, see Seifert, Komar, Barbosa et al., 2014).

In other chapters we have highlighted variables that describe sport performance by centring its discussion on kinematic and physiological performance indicators. It examines the application of these 'low level' performance indicators in sports, such as football, describing various methods that have been used to investigate the kinematic and physiological demands of sports. It describes the representativeness of combining accurate and reliable time–motion kinematical analysis, such as the position of players in the field or their body pose, with physiological indicators, so as to provide a more comprehensive understanding of the athletic performance.

Technological advances are a window of opportunity to further study and augment the understanding of the athletic performance. The material in this book seeks to provide a guide for setting up the analysis design, with emphasis on team sports, defining the task, the procedures, and relevant technology. It highlights the use of automated tools for assisting the behavioural analysis of performance in collective sports to make the difference in improving the individual and collective outcomes. It explains how to prepare and build the methodological setup to analyse athletic performance, considering the performance indicators described in the previous chapter. Several methodological and technological alternatives are presented and compared, with multiple case studies provided by the authors and applied to different sports. Among the multiple technologies surveyed, it covers traditional cameras, smartphones, TV broadcast tracking systems, 3D depth cameras, motion capture suits (optokinetic cameras and inertial measurement unit, smartwatches, and GPS), and sport-specific devices, supporting the design in both research and practice.

There is a need to continue to discover 'high level' performance indicators, or metrics, computed on top of the kinematic and physiological variables that are of interest to coaches, trainers, sport scientists, and athletes. Artificial intelligence enables sport practitioners to combine 'low level' indicators in 'high level' indicators that inform an understanding of movement coordination or provide insights through advanced metrics (e.g., complexity, entropy, resilience) that support the further exploitation of the meaning of 'low level' indicators. For instance, stride frequency or stroke rate in cyclic activities (e.g., running, rowing, arm and leg actions in swimming) exemplifies 'low level' indicators that can help explain changes in speed, since speed is a product of frequency and length of limb actions (striding or pulling with the arms). However, tracking, using motion capture systems, allows sport practitioners to obtain cycle-to-cycle data that can be modelled through the entire event/race in order to interpret and understand its variability (for an example of swimming speed in 50, 100, and 200 m front crawl race analysis, see Simbaña-Escobar, Hellard, & Seifert, 2018b; Simbaña-Escobar, Hellard, Pyne, & Seifert, 2018a). Several metrics that have been used to capture players' performance are described and algorithmically delineated, including individual metrics, such as the fractional-order coefficient of a player's trajectory, collective metrics, such as the effective area of play of the team, and network-related metrics, such as microscopic, mesoscopic, and macroscopic network measures. Every metric is illustrated, and their representativeness discussed, through multiple examples. These metrics have been used as features of the pattern recognition architectures presented in the book.

Another important contribution of the book is a survey of the current research directions of pattern recognition in sports by resorting to multiple classification methods, including support vector machines and multiple neural network approaches, such as faster regions with convolutional neural networks and long-short term memory networks. In the book, we analyse the use of these artificial intelligence methods to autonomously recognize actions and performance signatures, at both individual and collective levels, presenting their advantages and drawbacks, performance metrics required as representative features, and usage examples. Later chapters also discuss the research challenges, such as the individual profile of the athletes, especially at the physiological level, and technical limitations, as well as the remaining open research questions. The aim is to consider multiple examples, from individual to collective sports, with a particular emphasis in football.

The problem of modelling sports with the purpose of estimating performance characteristics that lead an athlete to succeed or not and a team to lose or win a match is also faced. However, behavioural (movement and coordination of movements) analyses may not reflect key performance outcomes' analyses (like scoring points, runs, or goals in competition) and vice versa. Moreover, modelling could be used for different functions like prediction or understanding, and could be undertaken at different time scales (a performance event such as race or game, a competitive season, or even over several seasons) and at different levels of analysis (micro-, meso-, and macro-; Clemente, Martins, & Mendes, 2016). For that purpose, it takes into consideration the contributions presented in some chapters to move from classification, through explanation, to prediction, with the intent to estimate various parameters that highly influence the functioning of a performance environment, including athlete's position, actions, and muscle fatigue. This approach led to the proposal of a novel sport prediction model, through which deep learning is used as a learning strategy. Additionally, we delineated the limitations inherent to several performance prediction approaches presented in the book. There is an attempt to present the implications of current approaches to performance prediction and consider the future endeavours they may lead to, whether in research, education, or training contexts.

Looking Ahead

In sport, increased accessibility and mobility of new technologies and related systems has led to a growing interest in their application to develop athlete performance. However, despite the number of sports organizations investing in advanced analytic systems, there is a need for more scientific evidence to inform and underpin their application in understanding sport performance and preparing and developing athletes of the future. Furthermore, the COVID-19 pandemic isolation of 2020–2021 has highlighted the opportunities and needs for remote coaching and athlete support, using information from digital technologies in sport. This is particularly the case for large-scale geographical locations such as North and South Americas, Australia, the European Union, Russia, China, and India, areas with often large distances between coaches, trainers, support staff, and athletes. At the same time, developing athletes have had access to digital tools for feedback and learning for a number of decades. What remains unclear is the appropriate use of technologies for different applications. Moreover, at the elite level, the use of machine learning, development of artificial intelligence, and computer vision in sport are beginning to create complex levels of feedback and analysis for coaches and sport practitioners. This complexity occurs because, with the development of technologies and algorithms, data analysts can undertake real-time analyses, delivering the capacity to provide rapid feedback during a competitive event. Therefore, AI is routinely used in a competitive event. To enable the full potential of these digital technologies in enhancing athlete performance and development in sport, a theoretical framework is necessary to rationalize applications of such systems to ensure effective and efficient designs of learning environments. As Stone and colleagues (2018) proposed, key concepts in ecological dynamics (i.e., an integration of concepts from ecological psychology, dynamic systems theory, complexity sciences, constraints-led practice, and representative learning design) can inform the design and the application of digital technologies to enable effective use of current and new technologies in supporting performance preparation and athlete development.

It is clear that there are different drivers of performance depending on the sport and the learner (Magill & Anderson, 2016). Surprisingly, motor learning and performance analysis have not yet been brought together in a structured approach to understanding how digital technologies can best fit needs. In other areas, such as the use of data mining in sport, researchers have created frameworks that consider matching the demands of the sport with the appropriate analysis and data mining methods (Ofoghi, Zeleznikow, MacMahon, & Raab, 2013). The link between skill acquisition practice and digital technologies is lacking, however. With regard to technology, there are three overarching questions for sport development and coaching:

1   What technologies are available for coaching, and do they align with both the big questions coaches ask, and motor learning principles?
2   How does the evolution of technology drive evolution in coaching practice, and vice versa?
3   In what ways are the universal coaching needs and interests represented in the drive for innovation in sports technology?

Framing the research with these key questions, this book provides information for those who seek to understand the use of digital technology in enhancing training and performance in sport. Sport training and performance have been undoubtedly enhanced by digital technologies. Not only do coaches have access to analysis and data as never before, but developing and experienced athletes alike can access performance and learning feedback. In large land masses like Australia, China, the Americas, and the European Union, technology provides a platform for high-level remote coaching. At developing levels, athletes can use a variety of platforms for disseminating AI, such as phone apps, instrumented equipment, and virtual reality. At elite levels, advances in computer vision provide unrivalled depth of information for coaches. In addition, however, the appropriate use of technologies can present a challenge and in some cases a paradox of choice (Schwartz, 2004), wherein the many options or ways of using technology may result in fraught decision analysis and dissatisfaction with the selection made. This project will seek to bridge the gap between the technologies and information available, and the skill learning principles for their effective use. However this book also emphasizes that the support (development and preparation) work of practitioners should not be merely 'data-driven' but should be 'data-informed'. Access to large sets of performance and training data is not intended to replace human decision-making by support staff functioning in a Department of Methodology. Rather data access should be considered as helpful to support practitioner decision-making in such organizations (Couceiro et al., 2016; Rothwell et al., 2020). The book sought to understand the appropriate application of different technologies, from simple filming and feedback, to virtual reality, computer vision, and deep learning, for coaches and athletes in developing and refining movement – general, and sport-specific skills.

The fast-paced development of emerging digital technologies creates exciting opportunities for cutting-edge innovation to address contemporary societal-level issues and transform lives. Maintaining and improving physical and mental health are major global concerns, and physical activity (PA) is widely acknowledged as a determining factor in ensuring physical, psychological, and emotional well-being. A shift towards home-based, indoor exercise is being driven by increasing urbanization and, more recently, by the worldwide pandemic that has enforced restrictions on movement outside of the home. Importantly, evidence suggests that exercise environments have an effect on the quality of PA (Yeh et al., 2016).

While traditional PA interventions consist of delivering regular individual and group-based behaviour change initiatives which can be costly, AI-assisted new and emerging digital technologies such as augmented reality (AR) and virtual reality (VR) can be used remotely and connect people over large distances or those with restricted travel. However, empirical research examining how to effectively design and implement VR during sport and physical activity is still limited (Stone et al., 2018). Recent attempts to implement VR technology in an exercise context have shown that the immersive qualities of the VR can create a pleasant and enjoyable exercise experience (Jones & Ekkekakis, 2019). Creating engaging and enjoyable exercise experiences is crucial for long-term adherence to exercise. By meaningfully engaging with potential users of emerging digital technologies, not only about the barriers they face, but about the types of strategies that would seek to reduce these barriers, the content and design of technologies such as virtual reality would likely be more effective. Therefore, a co-design approach to content design is essential and will guide organised programmes of physical activity.

In summary, the enrichment of physical activity through emerging digital technology offers a wealth of opportunities to acquire new skills, build communities among exercisers, create motivational environments, and ultimately transform lives. Therefore, a key intended outcome of this book has been to to examine the role of emerging digital technologies in enriching physical activity through, first, understanding the barriers associated with such technologies, and then to develop strategies to overcome those barriers with the aim of improving physical, mental, and emotional well-being in older adults.

The benefits of regular physical activity are widely acknowledged, but challenges remain as to how more people can achieve the recommended amount of physical activity per week. Physical activity targets worldwide are similar (e.g., UK and Australia recommend 150 minutes of moderate intensity activity, or 75 minutes of vigorous intensity activity, in addition to two strengthening activities per week), and prevalence of physical inactivity remains at 33% in the UK, and 55% in Australia. As the UK and Australia have ageing populations, the issues relating to physical inactivity of older adults will have a more immediate impact on society than inactivity of younger adults. Hence, the challenges faced by an ageing population are described in the UK government's Industrial Strategy, and it is accompanied by a call for new technologies to address these challenges.

The older adult population (50–64 years) are homogeneous in terms of age but face different barriers to engagement with exercise. The challenge is to understand the core issues underlying the barriers limiting people's engagement with exercise and to co-create effective content and strategies using emerging digital technologies to help address these barriers. For example, physical distance provides a barrier to exercise in Australia and interaction with other people is often not easy, whereas time to travel to exercise facilities is a barrier in the UK. Creating digital content to facilitate social interactions, in a format suitable for older adults, might address underlying issues present in both barriers to exercise while promoting the social support which is a powerful vehicle for motivation and engagement with exercise. Further, strength training is often the 'forgotten' physical activity recommendation and appropriately developed content through digital platforms could help older adults maintain strength through participation in physical activities and games. Play is important at all ages and could also help older adults to maintain movement capacities to safely engage in strengthening exercises to reduce frailty.

To realize the full potential of digital technology in enhancing physical activity, a theoretical framework is necessary to rationalize applications of such systems to ensure effective and efficient designs for the population group. Davids, Araújo, and Brymer (2016) discuss how the theoretical framework of ecological dynamics, specially the key concept of affordances (opportunities for action), can be used to regulate environmental interactions providing a basis for (re)designing PA and exercise contexts. By manipulating task constraints in specific environments, we can co-create affordances to help different population groups gain what they need when regulating their activities. Designing affordances into PA environments can 'nudge' individuals towards particular outcomes. As they emerge, behaviours can underpin each individual's structural (physical conditioning, agility, flexibility, and strength) and functional (cognitions, emotions, and fatigue reduction) needs in a specific environment. For example, the enjoyment of exercise is cited as a motivator for exercise, but a lack of enjoyment derived from exercise is a barrier. Engaging digital technologies (head-mounted displays) have been shown to increase the pleasure during exercise (Jones & Ekkekakis, 2019), but additional research is required to develop suitable content for an older adult population. Therefore, a key aim of future research is to engage with inactive older adults to understand the barriers they face to exercise and gain knowledge on how emerging digital technologies can be implemented to address these barriers.

REFERENCES

Abdel-Aziz, Y., & Karara, H. (1971). Direct linear transformation: From comparator coordinates into object coordinates in close range photogrammetry. In *Proceedings of the Symposium on Close-Range Photogrammetry* (pp. 1–18). Church Falls, VA: American Society of Photogrammetry.

Adjerid, I., & Kelley, K. (2018). Big data in psychology: A framework for research advancement. *American Psychologist, 73*, 899–917.

Adolph, K. E. (2016). Video as data: From transient behavior to tangible recording. *APS Observer, 29*, 23–25.

Agatonovic-Kustrin, S., & Beresford, R. (2000). Basic concepts of artificial neural network(ann) modeling and its application in pharmaceutical research. *Journal of Pharmaceutical and Biomedical Analysis, 22*(5), 717–727.

Aghajanzadeh, S., Jebb, A., Li, Y., Lu, Y-H., & Thiruvathukal, G. (2020). Observing human behavior through worldwide network cameras. In S. Woo, L. Tay, & R. Proctor (Eds.), *Big data in psychological research* (pp. 109–124). Washington, DC: American Psychological Association.

Ahmadi, A., Rowlands, D. D., & James, D. A. (2010). Development of inertial and novel marker-based techniques and analysis for upper arm rotational velocity measurements in tennis. *Sports Engineering, 12*(4), 179–188. doi:10.1007/s12283-010-0044-1.

Al Alwani, A. S., & Chahir, Y. (2016). Spatiotemporal representation of 3D skeleton joints-based action recognition using modified spherical harmonics. *Pattern Recognition Letters, 83*, 32–41. doi:10.1016/J.PATREC.2016.05.032.

Albert, R., Jeong, H., & Barabási, A. L. (2000). Error and attack tolerance in complex system. *Nature, 406*, 378. doi:10.1038/35019019.

Alexander, D. L., & Kern, W. (2005). Drive for show and putting for dough?: An analysis of the earnings of PGA tour golfers. *Journal of Sports Economics, 6*(1), 46–60. doi:10.1177/1527002503260797.

Alpaydin, E. (2009). *Introduction to machine learning.* Cambridge, MA: MIT Press.

Araújo, D., Brymer, E., Brito, H., Withagen, R., & Davids, K. (2019). The empowering variability of affordances of nature: Why do exercisers feel better after performing the same exercise in natural environments than in indoor environments? *Psychology of Sport & Exercise, 42,* 138–145.

Araújo, D., Cordovil, R., Ribeiro, J., Davids, K., & Fernandes, O. (2009). How does knowledge constrain sport performance? An ecological perspective. In D. Araújo, H. Ripoll, & M. Raab (Eds.), *Perspectives on cognition and action in sport* (pp. 100–120). Hauppauge, NY: Nova Science Publishers.

Araújo, D., & Davids, K. (2015). Towards a theoretically – driven model of correspondence between behaviours in one context to another: Implications for studying sport performance. *International Journal of Sport Psychology, 46,* 268–280.

Araújo, D., & Davids, K. (2016). Team synergies in sport: Theory and measures. *Frontiers in Psychology, 7,* 1449. doi:10.3389/fpsyg.2016.01449.

Araújo, D., & Davids, K. (2018). The (sport) performer-environment system as the base unit in explanations of expert performance. *Journal of Expertise, 1*(3), 144–154.

Araújo, D., Davids, K., & Hristovski, R. (2006). The ecological dynamics of decision making in sport. *Psychology of Sport and Exercise, 7,* 653–676.

Araújo, D., Davids, K., & Passos, P. (2007). Ecological validity, representative design, and correspondence between experimental task constraints and behavioral setting: Comment on Rogers, Kadar, and Costall (2005). *Ecological Psychology, 19*(1), 69–78.

Araújo, D., Davids, K., & Renshaw, I. (2020). Cognition, emotion and action in sport: An ecological dynamics perspective. In G. Tenenbaum & R. Eklund (Eds.), *Handbook of sport psychology* (4th ed., pp. 535–555). New York, NY: John Wiley & Sons, Inc.

Araújo, D., Davids, K., & Serpa, S. (2005). An ecological approach to expertise effects in decision-making in a simulated sailing regatta. *Psychology of Sport and Exercise, 6*(6), 671–692. doi:10.1016/j.psychsport.2004.12.003.

Araújo, D., Dicks, M., & Davids, K. (2019). Selecting among affordances: A basis for channeling expertise in sport. In M. L. Cappuccio (Ed.), *The MIT press handbook of embodied cognition and sport psychology* (pp. 557–580). Cambridge, MA: MIT Press.

Araújo, D., Diniz, A., Passos, P., & Davids, K. (2014). Decision making in social neurobiological systems modeled as transitions in dynamic pattern formation. *Adaptive Behaviour, 22*(1), 21–30.

Araújo, D., Fonseca, C., Davids, K. W., Garganta, J., Volossovitch, A., Brandão, R., & Krebs, R. (2010). The role of ecological constraints on expertise development. *Talent Development and Excellence, 2*(2), 165–179.

Araújo, D., Hristovski, R., Seifert, L., Carvalho, J., & Davids, K. (2019). Ecological cognition: Expert decision-making behaviour in sport. *International Review of Sport and Exercise Psychology, 12,* 1–25. doi:10.1080/1750984X.2017.1349826.

Arnason, A., Sigurdsson, S. B., Gudmundsson, A., Holme, I., Engebretsen, L., & Bahr, R. (2004). Physical fitness, injuries, and team performance in soccer. *Medicine & Science in Sports & Exercise, 36*(2), 278–285.

Arndt, C., & Brefeld, U. (2016). Predicting the future performance of soccer players. *Statistical Analysis and Data Mining, 9*(5), 373–382. doi:10.1002/sam.11321.

Aujouannet, Y. A., Bonifazi, M., Hintzy, F., Vuillerme, N., & Rouard, A. H. (2006). Effects of a high-intensity swim test on kinematic parameters in high-level athletes. *Applied Physiology, Nutrition, and Metabolism, 31*(2), 150–158. doi: 10.1139/h05-012.

Bacic, B., & Hume, P. A. (2018). Computational intelligence for qualitative coaching diagnostics: Automated assessment of tennis swings to improve performance and safety. *Big Data, 6*(4), 291–304. doi:10.1089/big.2018.0062.

Baker, J., & Farrow, D. (Eds.) (2015). *Routledge handbook of sport expertise*. London, UK: Routledge.

Baranski, P., & Strumillo, P. (2012). Enhancing positioning accuracy in urban terrain by fusing data from a GPS receiver, inertial sensors, stereo-camera and digital maps for pedestrian navigation. *Sensors, 12*(6), 6764–6801. doi:10.3390/s120606764.

Barber, D. (2012). *Bayesian reasoning and machine learning*. Cambridge, UK: Cambridge University Press.

Barris, S., & Button, C. (2008). A review of vision-based motion analysis in sport. *Sports Medicine, 38*(12), 1025–1043.

Barron, D., Ball, G., Robins, M., & Sunderland, C. (2018). Artificial neural networks and player recruitment in professional soccer. *Plos One, 13*(10). doi:10.1371/journal.pone.0205818.

Bartlett, R. (2014). *Introduction to sports biomechanics: Analysing human movement patterns*. New York, NY: Routledge.

Basmajian, J. V. (1962). Muscles alive. Their functions revealed by electromyography. *Academic Medicine, 37*(8), 802.

Beal, R., Norman, T. J., & Ramchurn, S. D. (2019). Artificial intelligence for team sports: A survey. *The Knowledge Engineering Review, 34*, e28.

Bellman, R. (1966). Dynamic programming. *Science, 153*(3731), 34–37.

Benezeth, Y., Jodoin, P.-M., Saligrama, V., & Rosenberger, C. (2009). Abnormal events detection based on spatio-temporal co-occurences. *2009 IEEE Conference on Computer Vision and Pattern Recognition* (pp. 2458–2465). doi:10.1109/CVPR.2009.5206686

Ben-Hur, A., & Weston, J. (2010). A user's guide to support vector machines. In *Data mining techniques for the life sciences* (pp. 223–239). New York, NY: Humana Press.

Bergeron, M. F., Landset, S., Maugans, T. A., Williams, V. B., Collins, C. L., Wasserman, E. B., & Khoshgoftaar, T. M. (2019). Machine learning in modeling high school sport concussion symptom resolve. *Medicine & Science in Sports & Exercise, 51*(7), 1362–1371. doi:10.1249/mss.0000000000001903.

Berman, D. H., & Hafner, C. D. (1989). The potential of artificial intelligence to help solve the crisis in our legal system. *Communications of the ACM, 32*(8), 928–938.

Bernardina, G. R., Cerveri, P., Barros, R. M., Marins, J. C., & Silvatti, A. P. (2016). Action sport cameras as an instrument to perform a 3D underwater motion analysis. *PLoS One, 11*(8), e0160490. doi:10.1371/journal.pone.0160490.

Bernardina, G. R., Cerveri, P., Barros, R. M., Marins, J. C., & Silvatti, A. P. (2017). In-air versus underwater comparison of 3D reconstruction accuracy using action sport cameras. *Journal of Biomechanics, 51*, 77–82. doi:10.1016/j.jbiomech.2016.11.068.

Bhalchandra, P., Deshmukh, N., Lokhande, S., & Phulari, S. (2009). A comprehensive note on complexity issues in sorting algorithms. *Advances in Computational Research, 1*(2), 1–9.

Bhandari, I., Colet, E., Parker, J., Pines, Z., Pratap, R., & Ramanujam, K. (1997). Advanced scout: Data mining and knowledge discovery in NBA data. *Data Mining and Knowledge Discovery, 1*(1), 121–125. doi:10.1023/a:1009782106822.

Bianchi, F., Facchinetti, T., & Zuccolotto, P. (2017). Role revolution: Towards a new meaning of positions in basketball. *Electronic Journal of Applied Statistical Analysis, 10*(3), 712–734. doi:10.1285/i20705948v10n3p712.

Bishop, C. M. (2006). *Pattern recognition and machine learning*. Berlin, Germany: Springer.

Blake, A., Lee, D., Rosa, R., & Sherman, R. (2020). Wearable cameras, machine vision, and big data analytics: Insights into people and the places they go. In S. Woo,

L. Tay, R. Proctor (Eds.), *Big data in psychological research* (pp. 125–144). Washington, DC: American Psychological Association.

Bland, J. M., & Altman, D. G. (1986). Statistical methods for assessing agreement between two methods of clinical measurement. *Lancet, 1*(8476), 307–310. doi:10.1016/S0140-6736(86)90837-8.

Bock, J. R. (2017). Empirical prediction of turnovers in NFL football. *Sports, 5*(1). doi:10.3390/sports5010001.

Boon, B. H., & Sierksma, G. (2003). Team formation: Matching quality supply and quality demand. *European Journal of Operational Research, 148*(2), 277–292.

Bostrom, N. (2017/2014). *Superintelligence. Paths, dangers, strategies.* Oxford, UK: Oxford University Press.

Bourbousson, J., Poizat, G., Saury, J., & Seve, C. (2010). Team coordination in basketball: Description of the cognitive connections among teammates. *Journal of Applied Sport Psychology, 22*(2), 150–166.

Bourbousson, J., Sève, C., & McGarry, T. (2010). Space–time coordination dynamics in basketball: Part 2. The interaction between the two teams. *Journal of Sports Sciences, 28*(3), 349–358.

Bouziane, A., Chahir, Y., Molina, M., & Jouen, F. (2013). Unified framework for human behaviour recognition: An approach using 3D Zernike moments. *Neurocomputing, 100*, 107–116. doi:10.1016/J.NEUCOM.2011.12.042.

Brandt, M., & Brefeld, U. (2015). Graph-based approaches for analyzing team interaction on the example of soccer. In *Machine Learning and Data Mining for Sports Analytics (MLSA15), European conference on machine learning and principles and practice of knowledge discovery in databases (ECML PKDD)* (pp. 10–17), Porto, Portugal.

Brent, R. P. (1973). *Algorithms for minimization without derivatives.* Englewood Cliffs, NJ: Prentice-Hall.

Brewin, M. A., & Kerwin, D. G. (2003). Accuracy of scaling and DLT reconstruction techniques for planar motion analyses. *Journal of Applied Biomechanics, 19*(1), 79–88.

Brooks, J., Kerr, M., & Guttag, J. (2016). Using machine learning to draw inferences from pass location data in soccer. *Statistical Analysis and Data Mining, 9*(5), 338–349. doi:10.1002/sam.11318.

Brumatti, M. (2005). *Redes neurais artificiais.* Espírito Santo: Vitória.

Brunelli, R., & Poggio, T. (1993). Face recognition: Features versus templates. *IEEE Transactions on Pattern Analysis and Machine Intelligence, 15*(10), 1042–1052.

Brunswik, E. (1956). *Perception and the representative design of psychological experiments* (2nd ed.). Berkeley: University of California Press.

Burdet, E., Tee, K. P., Mareels, I., Milner, T. E., Chew, C. M., Franklin, D. W., Osu, R., & Kawato, M. (2006). Stability and motor adaptation in human arm movements. *Biological Cybernetics, 94*(1), 20–32. doi:10.1007/s00422-005-0025-9.

Burrell, J. (2016). How the machine 'thinks': Understanding opacity in machine learning algorithms. *Big Data & Society, 3*(1), 1–12. doi:10.1177/2053951715622512.

Button, C., Seifert, L., Chow, J. Y., Araújo, D., & Davids, K. (2020). *Dynamics of skill acquisition: An ecological dynamics approach* (2nd ed.). Champaign, IL: Human Kinetics.

Byvatov, E., Fechner, U., Sadowski, J., & Schneider, G. (2003). Comparison of support vector machine and artificial neural network systems for drug/nondrug classification. *Journal of Chemical Information and Computer Sciences, 43*(6), 1882–1889.

Cai, Y., Wu, S., Zhao, W., Li, Z., Wu, Z., & Ji, S. (2018). Concussion classification via deep learning using whole-brain white matter fiber strains. *Plos One, 13*(5), e0197992. doi:10.1371/journal.pone.0197992.

Campaniço, A. T., Valente, A., Serôdio, R., & Escalera, S. (2018). Data's hidden data: Qualitative revelations of sports efficiency analysis brought by neural network performance metrics. *Motricidade, 14*(4), 94–102. doi:10.6063/motricidade.15984.

Campo, M., Champely, S., Lane, A. M., Rosnet, E., Ferrand, C., & Louvet, B. (2019). Emotions and performance in rugby. *Journal of Sport and Health Science, 8*(6), 595–600.

Cao, Z., Hidalgo, G., Simon, T., Wei, S. E., & Sheikh, Y. (2018). Openpose: realtime multi-person 2D pose estimation using part affinity fields. arXiv preprint arXiv:1812.08008.

Carling, C., Bloomfield, J., Nelsen, L., & Reilly, T. (2008). The role of motion analysis in elite soccer. *Sports Medicine, 38*(10), 839–862.

Carling, C., Bradley, P., McCall, A., & Dupont, G. (2016). Match-to-match variability in high-speed running activity in a professional soccer team. *Journal of Sports Sciences, 34*(24), 2215–2223.

Carrilho, D., Couceiro, M. S., Brito, J., Figueiredo, P., Lopes, R. J., & Araújo, D. (2020). Using optical tracking system data to measure team synergic behavior: Synchronization of player-ball-goal angles in a football match. *Sensors, 20*(17), 4990.

Carse, B., Meadows, B., Bowers, R., & Rowe, P. (2013). Affordable clinical gait analysis: An assessment of the marker tracking accuracy of a new low-cost optical 3D motion analysis system. *Physiotherapy, 99*(4), 347–351. doi:10.1016/j.physio.2013.03.001.

Ceccon, S., Ceseracciu, E., Sawacha, Z., Gatta, G., Cortesi, M., Cobelli, C., & Fantozzi, S. (2013). Motion analysis of front crawl swimming applying CAST technique by means of automatic tracking. *Journal of Sports Sciences, 13*(3), 276–287. doi:10.1080/02640414.2012.729134.

Chaffin, D., Heidl, R., Hollenbeck, J. R., Howe, M., Yu, A., Voorhees, C., & Calantone, R. (2017). The promise and perils of wearable sensors in organizational research. *Organizational Research Methods, 20*, 3–31.

Chahir, Y., Djerioui, M., Brik, Y., & Ladjal, M. (2019, December). *Heart disease prediction using neighborhood component analysis and support vector machines.* Paper presented at the VIIIth International Workshop on Representation, analysis and recognition of shape and motion FroM Imaging data (RFMI 2019), Sidi Bou Said, Tunisia.

Chai, T., & Draxler, R. R. (2014). Root mean square error (RMSE) or mean absolute error (MAE)? – Arguments against avoiding RMSE in the literature. *Geoscientific Model Development, 7*(3), 1247–1250.

Chambers, R. M., Gabbett, T. J., & Cole, M. H. (2019). Validity of a microsensor-based algorithm for detecting scrum events in rugby union. *International Journal of Sports Physiology and Performance, 14*(2), 176–182. doi:10.1123/ijspp.2018–0222.

Chawla, S., Estephan, J., Gudmundsson, J., & Horton, M. (2017). Classification of passes in football matches using spatiotemporal data. *ACM Transactions on Spatial Algorithms and Systems, 3*(2), 6. doi:10.1145/3105576.

Chen, H.-T., Chou, C.-L., Tsai, W.-C., Lee, S.-Y., & Lin, B.-S. P. (2012). HMM-based ball hitting event exploration system for broadcast baseball video. *Journal of Visual Communication and Image Representation, 23*(5), 767–781. doi:10.1016/j.jvcir.2012.03.006.

Cheng, G., Zhang, Z., Kyebambe, M. N., & Kimbugwe, N. (2016). Predicting the outcome of NBA playoffs based on the maximum entropy principle. *Entropy, 18*(12). doi:10.3390/e18120450.

Cho, Y., Yoon, J., & Lee, S. (2018). Using social network analysis and gradient boosting to develop a soccer win-lose prediction model. *Engineering Applications of Artificial Intelligence, 72*, 228–240. doi:10.1016/j.engappai.2018.04.010.

Chollet, D., Chalies, S., & Chatard, J. C. (2000). A new index of coordination for the crawl: description and usefulness. *International Journal of Sports Medicine, 21*(1), 54–59. doi:10.1055/s-2000–8855.

Cintra, R. S., Velho, H. F., & Todling, R. (2011). Redes neurais artificiais na melhoria de desempenho de métodos de assimilação de dados: Filtro de Kalman. *Trends in Applied and Computational Mathematics, 11*(1), 29–39.

Clark, R. A., Pua, Y. H., Fortin, K., Ritchie, C., Webster, K. E., Denehy, L., & Bryant, A. L. (2012). Validity of the Microsoft Kinect for assessment of postural control. *Gait Posture, 36*, 372–377. doi:10.1016/j.gaitpost.2012.03.033.

Claudino, J. G., Capanema, D. O., de Souza, T. V., Serrao, J. C., Machado Pereira, A. C., & Nassis, G. P. (2019). Current approaches to the use of artificial intelligence for injury risk assessment and performance prediction in team sports: A systematic review. *Sports Medicine Open, 5*(1), 28. doi:10.1186/s40798-019-0202-3.

Clemente, F. M., Couceiro, M. S., Martins, F. M. L., & Mendes, R. S. (2014). Using network metrics to investigate football team players' connections: A pilot study. *Motriz: Revista de Educação Física, 20*(3), 262–271.

Clemente, F. M., Couceiro, M. S., Martins, F. M. L., & Mendes, R. S. (2015). Using network metrics in soccer: A macro-analysis. *Journal of Human Kinetics, 45*(1), 123–134.

Clemente, F. M., Couceiro, M. S., Martins, F. M., Mendes, R., & Figueiredo, A. J. (2013). Measuring tactical behaviour using technological metrics: Case study of a football game. *International Journal of Sports Science & Coaching, 8*(4), 723–739.

Clemente, F. M., Martins, F. M., & Mendes, R. S. (2016). *Social network analysis applied to team sports analysis.* Heidelberg, Germany: Springer-Verlag.

Clemente, F. M., Sequeiros, J. B., Correia, A., Silva, F. G., & Martins, F. M. L. (Eds.). (2018). Individual metrics to characterize the players. In *Computational metrics for soccer analysis: Connecting the dots* (pp. 15–31). Heidelberg, Germany: Springer.

Cliff, O. M., Lizier, J. T., Wang, X. R., Wang, P., Obst, O., & Prokopenko, M. (2013). Towards quantifying interaction networks in a football match. In Behnke, S., Veloso, M. Visser, A., & Xiong, R. (Eds.), *Robot soccer world cup* (pp. 1–12). Berlin, Germany: Springer.

Constantinou, A., & Fenton, N. (2017). Towards smart-data: Improving predictive accuracy in long-term football team performance. *Knowledge-Based Systems, 124*, 93–104. doi:10.1016/j.knosys.2017.03.005.

Corrêa, N. K., Lima, J. C. M. d., Russomano, T., & Santos, M. A. d. (2017). Development of a skateboarding trick classifier using accelerometry and machine learning. *Research on Biomedical Engineering, 33*(4), 362–369. doi:10.1590/2446-4740.04717.

Cortès, U., Sànchez-Marrè, M., Ceccaroni, L., R-Roda, I., & Poch, M. (2000). Artificial intelligence and environmental decision support systems. *Applied Intelligence, 13*(1), 77–91.

Couceiro, M. (2020). PatRecog – Pattern Recognition Framework. Retrieved from https://www.mathworks.com/matlabcentral/fileexchange/69113-patrecog-pattern-recognition-framework, MATLAB Central File Exchange. Accessed September 16, 2020.

Couceiro, M., Clemente, F., Dias, G., Mendes, P., Martins, F., & Mendes, R. (2014). On an entropy-based performance analysis in sports. *Proceedings International Electronic Conference on Entropy and Its Applications, 1*, 1–20.

Couceiro, M., Clemente, F., & Martins, F. (2013). Analysis of football player's motion in view of fractional calculus. *Open Physics, 11*(6), 714–723.

Couceiro, M. S., Araújo, A. G., & Pereira, S. C. (2015). InPutter: An engineered putter for on-the-fly golf putting analysis. *Sports Technology, 8*(1–2), 12–29.

Couceiro, M. S., Clemente, F. M., Martins, F. M., & Machado, J. A. T. (2014). Dynamical stability and predictability of football players: The study of one match. *Entropy, 16*(2), 645–674.

Couceiro, M. S., Dias, G., Araújo, D., & Davids, K. (2016). The ARCANE project: How an ecological dynamics framework can enhance performance assessment and prediction in football. *Sports Medicine, 46*(12), 1781–1786.

Couceiro, M. S., Dias, G., Martins, F. M., & Luz, J. M. A. (2012). A fractional calculus approach for the evaluation of the golf lip-out. *Signal, Image and Video Processing, 6*(3), 437–443.

Couceiro, M. S., Dias, G., Mendes, R., & Araújo, D. (2013). Accuracy of pattern detection methods in the performance of golf putting. *Journal of Motor Behavior, 45*(1), 37–53.

Couceiro, M. S., Figueiredo, C. M., Luz, J. M. A., & Delorme, M. J. (2014). Zombie infection warning system based on Fuzzy decision-making. In R. J. Smith (Ed.)., *Mathematical modelling of zombies* (p. 171). Ottawa, Canada: University of Ottawa Press.

Courneya, K. S., & Carron, A. V. (1992). The home advantage in sport competitions: A literature review. *Journal of Sport & Exercise Psychology, 14*(1), 13–27.

Cuesta-Vargas, A. I., Galán-Mercant, A., & Williams, J. M. (2010). The use of inertial sensors system for human motion analysis. *Physical Therapy Reviews, 15*(6), 462–473. doi:10.1179/1743288X11Y.0000000006.

Cummins, C., Orr, R., O'Connor, H., & West, C. (2013). Global positioning systems (GPS) and microtechnology sensors in team sports: A systematic review. *Sports Medicine, 43*(10), 1025–1042. doi:10.1007/s40279-013-0069-2.

Cunningham, P., & Delany, S. J. (2020). k-nearest neighbour classifiers. arXiv preprint arXiv:2004.04523.

Cutti, A. G., Giovanardi, A., Rocchi, L., & Davalli, A. (2006). A simple test to assess the static and dynamic accuracy of an inertial sensors system for human movement analysis [Paper presentation]. *2006 International Conference of the IEEE Engineering in Medicine and Biology Society* (pp. 5912–5915). doi:10.1109/IEMBS.2006.260705.

Dadashi, F., Crettenand, F., Millet, G. P., & Aminian, K. (2012). Front-crawl instantaneous velocity estimation using a wearable inertial measurement unit. *Sensors, 12,* 12927–12939. doi:10.3390/s121012927.

Dadashi, F., Crettenand, F., Millet, G. P., Seifert, L., Komar, J., & Aminian K. (2013). Automatic front-crawl temporal phase detection using adaptive filtering of inertial signals. *Journal of Sports Sciences, 31*(11), 1251–1260.

Dadashi, F., Millet, G. P., & Aminian, K. (2016). Front-crawl stroke descriptors variability assessment for skill characterisation. *Journal of Sports Sciences, 14*(15), 1405–1412. doi:10.1080/02640414.2015.1114134.

Davids, K., & Araújo, D. (2010). The concept of "Organismic asymmetry" in sport science. *Journal of Science and Medicine in Sport, 13*(6), 633–640.

Davids, K., Araújo, D., & Brymer, E. (2016). Designing affordances for health enhancing physical activity and exercise in sedentary individuals. *Sports Medicine, 46*(7), 933–938. doi:10.1007/s40279-016-0511-3.

Davids, K., Araújo, D., Hristovski, R., Passos, P., & Chow, J. Y. (2012). Ecological dynamics and motor learning design in sport. In N. J. Hodges & M. A. Williams (Eds.), *Skill acquisition in sport: Research, theory and practice* (pp. 112–130). New York, NY: Routledge.

Davids, K., Handford, C., & Williams, M. (1994). The natural physical alternative to cognitive theories of motor behaviour: An invitation for interdisciplinary research in sports science? *Journal of Sports Sciences, 12*, 495–528.

Davids, K., Hristovski, R., Araújo, D., Balague, N., Button, C., & Passos, P. (Eds.). (2014). *Complex systems in sport.* London, UK: Routledge.

Davids, K., & Wall, T. D. (1990). Advanced manufacturing technology and shop floor work organisation. *The Irish Journal of Psychology, 11*(2), 109–129. doi:10.1080/03033910. 1990.105577906.

de Jesus, K., de Jesus, K., Figueiredo, P., Vilas-Boas, J.-P., Fernandes, R. J., & Machado, L. J. (2015). Reconstruction accuracy assessment of surface and underwater 3D motion analysis: A new approach. *Computational and Mathematical Methods in Medicine, 2015*, 269264. doi:10.1155/2015/269264.

De Luca, C. J. (2002). Surface electromyography: Detection and recording. *DelSys Incorporated, 10*(2), 1–10.

de Magalhães, F. A., Giovanardi, A., Cortesi, M., Gatta, G., & Fantozzi, S. (2013, August). *Three-dimensional kinematic analysis of shoulder through wearable inertial and magnetic sensors during swimming strokes simulation.* Paper presented at the XXIV Congress of the International Society of Biomechanics, Natal, Brazil.

de Magalhães, F. A., Vannozzi, G., Gatta, G., & Fantozzi, S. (2015). Wearable inertial sensors in swimming motion analysis: A systematic review. *Journal of Sports Sciences, 33*(7), 732–745. doi:10.1080/02640414.2014.962574.

Delen, D., Cogdell, D., & Kasap, N. (2012). A comparative analysis of data mining methods in predicting NCAA bowl outcomes. *International Journal of Forecasting, 28*(2), 543–552. doi:10.1016/j.ijforecast.2011.05.002.

Dias, G., & Couceiro, M. S. (2015). *The science of golf putting: A complete guide for researchers, players and coaches.* London, UK: Springer.

Dicharry, J. (2010). Kinematics and kinetics of gait: From lab to clinic. *Clinics in Sports Medicine, 29*(3), 347–64.

Dicks, M., Button, C., & Davids, K. (2010). Examination of gaze behaviors under in situ and video simulation task constraints reveals differences in information pickup for perception and action. *Attention, Perception, & Psychophysics, 72*, 706–720.

Dogramac, S. N., Watsford, M. L., & Murphy, A. J. (2011). The reliability and validity of subjective notational analysis in comparison to GPS tracking to assess athlete movement patterns. *The Journal of Strength and Conditioning Research, 25*(3), 852–859.

Dooley, T., & Titz, C. (2010). *Soccer: 4-4-2 System.* Berlin, Germany: Meyer & Meyer Verlag.

Dreyfus, H. (1992). *What computers still can't do: A critique of artificial reason.* Cambridge, MA: MIT Press.

Dreyfus, H. (2007). Why Heideggerian ai failed and how fixing it would require making it more Heideggerian. *Philosophical Psychology, 20*, 247–268.

Duarte, R., Araújo, D., Correia, V., & Davids, K. (2012). Sports teams as superorganisms. *Sports Medicine, 42*(8), 633–642.

Duarte, R., Araújo, D., Correia, V., Davids, K., Marques, P., & Richardson, M. (2013). Competing together: Assessing the dynamics of team-team and player-team synchrony in professional football. *Human Movement Science, 2*, 555–566.

Duch, J., Waitzman, J. S., & Amaral, L. A. N. (2010). Quantifying the performance of individual players in a team activity. *PloS One, 5*(6), e10937. doi:10.1371/journal. pone.0010937.

Düking, P., Hotho, A., Holmberg, H. C., Fuss, F. K., & Sperlich, B. (2016). Comparison of non-invasive individual monitoring of the training and health of athletes with commercially available wearable technologies. *Frontiers in Physiology, 7,* 71.

Duthie, G., Pyne, D., & Hooper, S. (2003). The reliability of video based time motion analysis. *Journal of Human Movement Studies, 44,* 259–272.

Edwards, J. R., & Bagozzi, R. P. (2000). On the nature and direction of relationships between constructs and measures. *Psychological Methods, 5,* 155–174.

Ekstrand, J. (2013). Keeping your top players on the pitch: The key to football medicine at a professional level. *British Journal of Sports Medicine, 47*(12), 723–724. doi:10.1136/bjsports-2013-092771.

Elhoseny, M. (2020). Multi-object Detection and Tracking (MODT) machine learning model for real-time video surveillance systems. *Circuits, Systems, and Signal Processing, 39*(2), 611–630. doi:10.1007/s00034-019-01234-7.

Ellis, G., & Dix, A. (2006). An explorative analysis of user evaluation studies in information visualisation. In E. Bertini, C. Plaisant, & G. Santucci (Eds.), *Proceedings of the 2006 AVI workshop on beyond time and errors: Novel evaluation methods for information visualization* (pp. 1–7). New York, NY: ACM.

Endel, F., & Piringer, H. (2015). Data wrangling: Making data useful again. *International Federation of Automatic Control, 48,* 111–112.

Ericsson, A., Hoffman, R., Kozbelt, A., & Williams, M. (Eds.). (2018). *Cambridge handbook of expertise and expert performance* (2nd ed.). Cambridge, UK: Cambridge University Press.

Ertel, W. (2017). *Introduction to artificial intelligence.* Weingarten, Germany: Springer.

Fan, W., & Bifet, A. (2014). Mining big data: Current status, and forecast to the future. *ACM SIGKDD Explorations Newsletter, 16,* 1–5.

Fantozzi, S., Giovanardi, A., de Magalhães, F. A., Di Michele, R., Cortesi, M., & Gatta, G. (2016). Assessment of three-dimensional joint kinematics of the upper limb during simulated swimming using wearable inertial-magnetic measurement units. *Journal of Sports Sciences, 34*(11), 1073–1080. doi:10.1080/02640414.2015.1088659.

Faria, D. R., Premebida, C., & Nunes, U. (2014). A probabilistic approach for human everyday activities recognition using body motion from RGB-D images. In *The 23rd IEEE international symposium on robot and human interactive communication* (pp. 732–737). Edinburgh, Scotland: IEEE.

Ferreira, J. F., & Dias, J. M. (2014). *Probabilistic approaches to robotic perception.* Berlin, Germany: Springer International Publishing.

Figueiredo, P., Machado, L., Vilas-Boas, J. P., & Fernandes, R. J. (2011). Reconstruction error of calibration volume's coordinates for 3D swimming kinematics. *Journal of Human Kinetics, 29,* 35–40. doi:10.2478/v10078-011-0037-6.

Fink, P. W., Foo, P. S., & Warren, W. H. (2009). Catching fly balls in virtual reality: A critical test of the outfielder problem. *Journal of Vision, 9,* 14.

Fok, W. W., Chan, L. C., & Chen, C. (2018). Artificial intelligence for sport actions and performance analysis using recurrent neural network (RNN) with long short-term memory (LSTM). In *Proceedings of the 2018 4th international conference on robotics and artificial intelligence* (pp. 40–44).

Fonseca, S., Milho, J., Passos, P., Araújo, D., & Davids, K. (2012). Approximate entropy normalized measures for analyzing social neurobiological systems. *Journal of Motor Behavior, 44*(3), 179–183.

Fonseca, S. T., Souza, T. R., Verhagen, E., Van Emmerik, R., Bittencourt, N. F., Mendonça, L. D., Andrade, A. G. P., Resende, R. A., & Ocarino, J. M. (2020). Sports injury forecasting and complexity: A synergetic approach. *Sports Medicine, 50*(10), 1757–1770. doi:10.1007/s40279-020-01326-4.

Ford, M. (2013). Could artificial intelligence create an unemployment crisis? *Communications of the ACM, 56*(7), 37–39.

Forsythe, G. E., Malcolm, M. A., & Moler, C. B. (1977). *Computer methods for mathematical computations* (Vol. 259). Englewood Cliffs, NJ: Prentice-Hall.

Fortes, L. S., Lima-Júnior, D., Nascimento-Júnior, J. R. A., Costa, E. C., Matta, M. O., & Ferreira, M. E. C. (2019). Effect of exposure time to smartphone apps on passing decision-making in male soccer athletes. *Psychology of Sport and Exercise, 44*, 35–41.

Freeman, C. L. (1978). Centrality in social networks conceptual clarification. *Social Networks, 1*(3), 215–239.

Frencken, W., Lemmink, K., Delleman, N., & Visscher, C. (2011). Oscillations of centroid position and surface area of soccer teams in small-sided games. *European Journal of Sport Science, 11*(4), 215–223.

Frencken, W. G. P., & Lemmink, K. A. P. M. (2008). Team kinematics of small-sided soccer games: A systematic approach. In Reilly, T., & Korkusuz, F. (Eds.), *Science and football VI* (pp. 187–192). London, UK: Routledge.

Fukuda, T. Y., Echeimberg, J. O., Pompeu, J. E., Lucareli, P. R. G., Garbelotti, S., Gimenes, R. O., & Apolinário, A. (2010). Root mean square value of the electromyographic signal in the isometric torque of the quadriceps, hamstrings and brachial biceps muscles in female subjects. *The Journal of Applied Research, 10*(1), 32–39.

Furukawa, Y., & Ponce, J. (2010). Accurate dense, and robust multiview stereopsis. *IEEE Transactions on Pattern Analysis and Machine Intelligence, 32*(8), 1362–1376. doi:10.1109/TPAMI.2009.161

Gama, J., Couceiro, M., Dias, G., & Vaz, V. (2015). Small-world networks in professional football: Conceptual model and data. *European Journal of Human Movement, 35*, 85–113.

Gama, J., Dias, G., Passos, P., Couceiro, M., & Davids, K. (2020). Homogeneous distribution of passing between players of a team predicts attempts to shoot at goal in association football: A case study with 10 matches. *Nonlinear Dynamics, Psychology, and Life Sciences, 24*(3), 353–365.

Gama, J., Passos, P., Davids, K., Relvas, H., Ribeiro, J., Vaz, V., & Dias, G. (2014). Network analysis and intra-team activity in attacking phases of professional football. *International Journal of Performance Analysis in Sport, 14*(3), 692–708.

Gandomi, A., & Haider, M. (2015). Beyond the hype: Big data concepts, methods, and analytics. *International Journal of Information Management, 35*, 137–144.

Gao, Z., Yu, Y., Zhou, Y., & Du, S. (2015). Leveraging two kinect sensors for accurate full-body motion capture. *Sensors, 15*, 24297–24317. doi:10.3390/s150924297.

García, S., Luengo, J., & Herrera, F. (2016). Tutorial on practical tips of the most influential data preprocessing algorithms in data mining. *Knowledge-Based Systems, 98*, 1–29.

Geurkink, Y., Vandewiele, G., Lievens, M., de Turck, F., Ongenae, F., Matthys, S. P. J., Boone, J., & Bourgois, J. G. (2019). Modeling the prediction of the session rating of perceived exertion in soccer: Unraveling the puzzle of predictive indicators. *International Journal of Sports Physiology and Performance, 14*(6), 841–846. doi:10.1123/ijspp.2018-0698.

Gibson, J. J. (1979). *The ecological approach to visual perception*. Boston, MA: Houghton Mifflin.

Goddard, J., & Asimakopoulos, I. (2004). Forecasting football results and the efficiency of fixed-odds betting. *Journal of Forecasting, 23*(1), 51–66.

Goes, F., Meerhoff, L., Bueno, M., Rodrigues, D., Moura, F., Brink, M., Elferink-Gemser, M., Knobbe, A., Cunha, S., Torres, R., & Lemmink, K. (2020). Unlocking the potential of big data to support tactical performance analysis in professional soccer: A systematic review. *European Journal of Sport Science (online)*. doi:10.1080/17461391.2020.1747552.

Gomez, G., Herrera Lopez, P., Link, D., & Eskofier, B. (2014). Tracking of ball and players in beach volleyball videos. *Plos One, 9*(11), e111730. doi:10.1371/journal.pone.0111730.

Gourgoulis, V., Aggeloussis, N., Kasimatis, P., Vezos, N., Boli, A., & Mavromatis, G. (2008). Reconstruction accuracy in underwater three-dimensional kinematic analysis. *Journal of Science and Medicine in Sport, 11*(2), 90–95. doi:10.1016/j.jsams.2007.02.010.

Gowsikhaa, D., Abirami, S., & Baskaran, R. (2014). Automated human behavior analysis from surveillance videos: A survey. *Artificial Intelligence Review, 42*, 747–765.

Graupe, D. (2007). *Principles of artificial neural networks* (Vol. 6). Singapore: World Scientific.

Graves, A. (2012). Supervised sequence labelling. In *Supervised sequence labelling with recurrent neural networks* (pp. 5–13). Berlin, Heidelberg: Springer.

Graves, A. & Schmidhuber, J. (2005). Framewise phoneme classification with bidirectional lstm and other neural network architectures. *Neural Networks, 18*(5–6), 602–610.

Gray, A. J., Jenkins, D., Andrews, M. H. (2010). Validity and reliability of GPS for measuring distance travelled in field-based team sports. *Journal of Sports Sciences, 28*, 1319–1325.

Grehaigne, J. F. (1993). *L'organisation du jeu en football*. Paris: Éd. Action.

Grehaigne, J. F., Bouthier, D., & David, B. (1997). Dynamic-system analysis of opponent relationships in collective actions in soccer. *Journal of Sports Sciences, 15*(2), 137–149.

Grimm, K., Stegmann, G., Jacobucci, R., & Serang, S. (2020). Big data in developmental psychology. In S. Woo, L. Tay, & R. Proctor (Eds.), *Big data in psychological research* (pp. 297–318). Washington, DC: American Psychological Association.

Grunz, A., Memmert, D., & Perl, J. (2012). Tactical pattern recognition in soccer games by means of special self-organizing maps. *Human Movement Science, 31*(2), 334–343. doi:10.1016/j.humov.2011.02.008.

Guignard, B., Rouard, A., Chollet, D., Bonifazi, M., Dalla Vedova, D., Hart, J., & Seifert, L. (2020). Coordination dynamics of upper limbs in swimming: Effects of speed and fluid flow manipulation. *Research Quarterly for Exercise and Sport, 91*(3), 433–444. doi:10.1080/02701367.2019.1680787.

Guignard, B., Rouard, A., Chollet, D., Hart, J., Davids, K., & Seifert, L. (2017a). Individual-environment interactions in swimming: The smallest unit for analysing the emergence of coordination dynamics in performance? *Sports Medicine, 47*(8), 1543–1554. doi:10.1007/s40279-017-0684-4.

Guignard, B., Rouard, A., Chollet, D., & Seifert L. (2017b). Behavioral dynamics in swimming: The appropriate use of inertial measurement units. *Frontiers in Psychology, 8*, 383. doi:10.3389/fpsyg.2017.00383.

Güllich, A., Hardy, L., Kuncheva, L., Woodman, T., Laing, S., Barlow, M., Evans, L., Rees, T., Abernethy, B., Côté, J., Warr, C., & Wraith, L., (2019). Developmental biographies of olympic super-elite and elite athletes: A multidisciplinary pattern recognition analysis. *Journal of Expertise, 2*, 23–46.

Haider, S., Kaye-Kauderer, H. P., Maniya, A. Y., Dai, J. B., Li, A. Y., Post, A. F., Sobotka, S., Adams, R., Gometz, A., Lovell, M. R., & Choudhri, T. F. (2018). Does the environment influence they frequency of concussion incidence in professional football? *Cureus, 10*(11), e3627. doi:10.7759/cureus.3627.

Haig, B. (2020). Big data science: A philosophy of science perspective. In S. Woo, L. Tay, & R. Proctor (Eds.), *Big data in psychological research* (pp. 15–34). Washington, DC: American Psychological Association.

Harari, G. M., Lane, N. D., Wang, R., Crosier, B. S., Campbell, A. T., & Gosling, S. D. (2016). Using smartphones to collect behavioral data in psychological science: Opportunities, practical considerations, and challenges. *Perspectives on Psychological Science, 11*, 838–854.

Harrison, H. S., Turvey, M. T., & Frank, T. D. (2016). Affordance-based perception-action dynamics: A model of visually guided braking. *Psychological Review, 123*, 305–323.

Hausler, J., Halaki, M., & Orr, R. (2016). Application of global positioning system and microsensor technology in competitive rugby league match-play: A systematic review and meta-analysis. *Sports Medicine, 46*(4), 559–588. doi:10.1007/s40279-015-0440-6.

Hearst, M. A., Dumais, S. T., Osuna, E., Platt, J., & Scholkopf, B. (1998). Support vector machines. *IEEE Intelligent Systems and Their Applications, 13*(4), 18–28. doi:10.1109/5254.708428.

Heaven, W. (2020). Our weird behavior during the pandemic is messing with AI models. *MIT Technology Review.* Retrieved from https://www.technologyreview.com/2020/05/11/1001563/covid-pandemic-broken-ai-machine-learning-amazon-retail-fraud-humans-in-the-loop.

Heckerman, D. (1997). Bayesian networks for data mining. *Data Mining and Knowledge Discovery, 1*(1), 79–119.

Hopkins, W. G. (2000). Measures of reliability in sports medicine and science. *Sports Medicine, 30*, 1–15.

Horvath, S. (2011). *Weighted network analysis: Applications in genomics and systems biology.* London, UK: Springer.

Hsu, C.-C., Chen, H.-T., Chou, C.-L., & Lee, S.-Y. (2016). 2D Histogram-based player localization in broadcast volleyball videos. *Multimedia Systems, 22*(3), 325–341. doi:10.1007/s00530-015-0463-8.

Hughes, M., & Franks, I. (2004). *Notational analysis of sport: Systems for better coaching and performance in sport* (2nd ed.). London, UK: Routledge.

Hughes, M., & Franks, I. (2008). *The essentials of performance analysis: An introduction.* London, UK: Routledge.

Hughes, M., Franks, I. M., & Dancs, H. (Eds.). (2019). *Essentials of performance analysis in sport.* New York, NY: Routledge.

Ichikawa, H., Ohgi, Y., & Miyaji, C. (1998). Analysis of stroke of the freestyle swimming using an accelerometer. In K. Keskinen, P. Komi, & P. Hollander (Eds.), *Biomechanics and medicine in swimming VIII* (pp. 159–164). Jyväskylä, Finland: University of Jyväskylä.

Ida, H., Fukuhara, K., Sawada, M., & Ishii, M. (2011). Quantitative relation between server motion and receiver anticipation in tennis: Implications of responses to computer-simulated motions. *Perception*, *40*(10), 1221–1236. doi:10.1068/p7041.

Iskakov, K., Burkov, E., Lempitsky, V., & Malkov, Y. (2019). Learnable triangulation of human pose. *Proceedings of the IEEE international conference on computer vision* (pp. 7718–7727). doi:10.1109/ICCV.2019.00781.

Jackson, P. R., & Wall, T. D. (1991). How does operator control enhance performance of advanced manufacturing technology? *Ergonomics*, *34*(10), 1301–1311, doi:10.1080/00140139108964869.

Jaeger, J. M., & Schoellhorn, W. I. (2012). Identifying individuality and variability in team tactics by means of statistical shape analysis and multilayer perceptrons. *Human Movement Science*, *31*(2), 303–317. doi:10.1016/j.humov.2010.09.005.

Jäger, J. M., & Schöllhorn, W. I. (2007). Situation-orientated recognition of tactical patterns in volleyball. *Journal of Sports Sciences*, *25*(12), 1345–1353. Retrieved from http://search.ebscohost.com/login.aspx?direct=true&db=s3h&AN=26446998& lang=pt-pt&site=ehost-live&scope=site.

Jain, A. K., Mao, J., & Mohiuddin, K. M. (1996). Artificial neural networks: A tutorial. *Computer*, *29*(3), 31–44.

James, N. (2012). Predicting performance over time using a case study in real tennis. *Journal of Human Sport and Exercise*, *7*(2), 421–433. doi:10.4100/jhse.2012.72.08.

Jaspers, A., De Beeck, T. O., Brink, M. S., Frencken, W. G. P., Staes, F., Davis, J. J., & Helsen, W. F. (2018). Relationships between the external and internal training load in professional soccer: What can we learn from machine learning? *International Journal of Sports Physiology and Performance*, *13*(5), 625–630. doi:10.1123/ijspp.2017-0299.

Jennings, D., Cormack, S., Coutts, A. J., Boyd, L., & Aughey, R. J. (2010). The validity and reliability of GPS units for measuring distance in team sport specific running patterns. *International Journal of Sports Physiology and Performance*, *5*(3), 328–341. doi:10.1123/ijspp.5.3.328.

Jerritta, S., Murugappan, M., Nagarajan, R., & Wan, K. (2011). Physiological signals based human emotion recognition: A review. In *2011 IEEE 7th International Colloquium on Signal Processing and its Applications* (pp. 410–415). Penang, Malaysia: IEEE.

Jiang, C., Chen, Y., Chen, S., Bo, Y., Li, W., Tian, W., & Guo, J. (2019). A mixed deep recurrent neural network for MEMS gyroscope noise suppressing. *Electronics*, *8*(2), 181.

Johnston, R. J., Watsford, M. L., Pine, M. J., Spurrs, R. W., Murphy, A. J., & Pruyn, E. C. (2012). The validity and reliability of 5-Hz global positioning system units to measure team sport movement demands. *Journal of Strength and Conditioning Research*, *26*(3), 758–765. doi:10.1519/JSC.0b013e318225f161.

Jones, L., & Ekkekakis, P. (2019). Affect and prefrontal haemodynamics during exercise under immersive audiovisual stimulation: Improving the experience of exercise for overweight adults. *Journal of Sport & Health Science*, *8*(4), 325–38.

Jonsson, G. K., Anguera, M. T., Blanco-Villasenor, A., Losada, J. L., Hernandez-Mendo, A., Arda, T., Camerino, O., & Castellano, J. (2006). Hidden patterns of play interaction in soccer using SOF-CODER. *Behavior Research Methods*, *38*(3), 372–381. doi:10.3758/bf03192790.

Joseph, A., Fenton, N. E., & Neil, M. (2006). Predicting football results using Bayesian nets and other machine learning techniques. *Knowledge-Based Systems*, *19*(7), 544–553. doi:10.1016/j.knosys.2006.04.011.

Júdice, P., Magalhães, J., Rosa, G., Henriques-Neto, D., Hetherington-Rauth, M., & Sardinha, L. B. (2020, online). Sensor-based physical activity, sedentary time, and reported cell phone screen time: A hierarchy of correlates in youth. *Journal of Sport and Health Science.* doi:10.1016/j.jshs.2020.03.003.

Kampakis, S. (2013). Comparison of machine learning methods for predicting the recovery time of professional football players after an undiagnosed injury. In *MLSA@ PKDD/ECML* (pp. 58–68).

Karimzadeh, M., Zhao, J., Wang, G., Snyder, L., & Ebert, D. (2020). Human-guided visual analytics for big data. In S. Woo, L. Tay, & R. Proctor (Eds.), *Big data in psychological research* (pp. 145–178). Washington, DC: American Psychological Association.

Kazhdan, M., Bolitho, M., & Hoppe, H. (2006). Poisson surface reconstruction. *ACM International Conference Proceeding Series, 256,* 61–70.

Kellmann, M. (2010). Preventing overtraining in athletes in high-intensity sports and stress/recovery monitoring. *Scandinavian Journal of Medicine & Science in Sports, 20,* 95–102.

Kelly, D., Coughlan, G., Green, B., & Caulfield, B. (2012). Automatic detection of collisions in elite level rugby union using a wearable sensing device. *Sports Engineering (Springer Science & Business Media B.V.), 15*(2), 81–92. Retrieved from http://search.ebscohost.com/login.aspx?direct=true&db=s3h&AN=75253946&lang=pt-pt&site=ehost-live&scope=site.

Kempe, M., Grunz, A., & Memmert, D. (2015). Detecting tactical patterns in basketball: Comparison of merge self-organising maps and dynamic controlled neural networks. *European Journal of Sport Science, 15*(4), 249–255. doi:10.1080/17461391.2014.933882.

Kennedy, J. (2006). Swarm intelligence. In Zomaya, A. Y. (Ed.), *Handbook of nature-inspired and innovative computing* (pp. 187–219). Boston, MA: Springer.

Khillari, S. (2020). Artificial intelligence in manufacturing market size, share| Global Research Report, 2026.

Komar J., Seifert L., & Thouvarecq R. (2015). What variability tells us about motor expertise: Measurements and perspectives from a complex system approach. *Movement & Sport Sciences – Science & Motricité, 89,* 65–77.

Konrad, P. (2005). *A practical introduction to kinesiological electromyography.* Scottsdale, AZ: Noraxon INC.

Kovalchik, S., & Reid, M. (2018). A shot taxonomy in the era of tracking data in professional tennis. *Journal of Sports Sciences, 36*(18), 2096–2104. doi:10.1080/02640414.2018.1438094.

Kovalchik, S. A., Sackmann, J., & Reid, M. (2017). Player, official or machine?: Uses of the challenge system in professional tennis. *International Journal of Performance Analysis in Sport, 17*(6), 961–969. doi:10.1080/24748668.2017.1410340.

Kubat, M. (2015). *An introduction to machine learning.* Champ: Springer International Publishing.

Kugler, P. N., & Turvey, M. T. (1987). *Information, natural law, and the self-assembly of rhythmic movement.* Hillsdale, NJ: Lawrence Erlbaum Associates.

Kumar, E. P., & Sharma, E. P. (2014). Artificial neural networks – A study. *International Journal of Emerging Engineering Research and Technology, 2*(2), 143–148.

Kwon, Y. H. (1999). A camera calibration algorithm for the underwater motion analysis. In R. H. Sanders & B. J. Gibson (Eds.), *Proceedings of the XVIIth International Symposium on Biomechanics in Sports* (pp. 257–260). Perth, WA: Edith Cowan University.

Lai, M., Meo, R., Schifanella, R., & Sulis, E. (2018). The role of the network of matches on predicting success in table tennis. *Journal of Sports Sciences, 36*(23), 2691–2698. do i:10.1080/02640414.2018.1482813

Lake, D. E., Richman, J. S., Griffin, M. P., & Moorman, J. R. (2002). Sample entropy analysis of neonatal heart rate variability. *American Journal of Physiology-Regulatory, Integrative and Comparative Physiology, 283*(3), R789-R797.

Lam, M. W. Y. (2018). One-match-ahead forecasting in two-team sports with stacked bayesian regressions. *Journal of Artificial Intelligence and Soft Computing Research, 8*(3), 159–171. doi:10.1515/jaiscr-2018-0011.

Lapham, A. C., & Bartlett, R. M. (1995). The use of artificial intelligence in the analysis of sports performance: A review of applications in human gait analysis and future directions for sports biomechanics. *Journal of Sports Sciences, 13*(3), 229–237.

Lara Cueva, R. A., & Estevez Salazar, A. D. (2018). Towards an automatic detection system of sports talents: An approach to Tae Kwon Do. *Sistemas & Telematica, 16*(47), 31–44. doi:10.18046/syt.v16i47.3213.

Lassoued, I., Zagrouba, E., & Chahir, Y. (2016). A new approach of action recognition based on Motion Stable Shape (MSS) features. *2016 IEEE/ACS 13th International Conference of Computer Systems and Applications (AICCSA) (IEEE)*, 1–8. doi:10.1109/AICCSA.2016.7945652.

LeCun, Y., Bengio, Y., & Hinton, G. (2015). Deep learning. *Nature, 521*, 436–444.

Lee, L., & Grimson, W. E. L. (2002). Gait analysis for recognition and classification. In *Proceedings of fifth IEEE international conference on automatic face gesture recognition* (pp. 155–162). Washington, DC: IEEE.

Leicht, A. S., Gomez, M. A., & Woods, C. T. (2017). Team performance indicators explain outcome during women's basketball matches at the olympic games. *Sports, 5*(4). doi:10.3390/sports5040096.

Leite, W. S. (2017). Home advantage: Comparison between the major European football leagues. *Athens Journal of Sports, 4*(1), 65–74.

Leo, M., Mazzeo, P. L., Nitti, M., & Spagnolo, P. (2013). Accurate ball detection in soccer images using probabilistic analysis of salient regions. *Machine Vision and Applications, 24*(8), 1561–1574. doi:10.1007/s00138-013-0518-9.

Li, E. Y. (1994). Artificial neural networks and their business applications. *Information & Management, 27*(5), 303–313.

Liang, K., Chahir, Y., Molina, M., Tijus, C., & Jouen, F. (2014). Appearance-based eye control system by manifold learning. *Proceedings of the 9th international conference on computer vision theory and applications – volume 3: VISAPP* (pp. 148–155). Lisbon, Portugal: IEEE. doi:10.5220/0004682601480155.

Liddy, J. J., Zelaznik, H. N., Huber, J. E., Rietdyk, S., Claxton, L. J., Samuel, A., & Haddad, J. M. (2017). The efficacy of the Microsoft KinectTM to assess human bimanual coordination. *Behaviour Research Methods, 49*(3), 1030–1047. doi:10.3758/s13428-016-0764-7.

Lim, S. M., Oh, H. C., Kim, J., Lee, J., & Park, J. (2018). LSTM-guided coaching assistant for table tennis practice. *Sensors (Basel), 18*(12). doi:10.3390/s18124112.

Link, D., & Hoernig, M. (2017). Individual ball possession in soccer. *Plos ONE, 12*(7), e0179953. doi:10.1371/journal.pone.0179953.

Linke, D., Link, D., & Lames, M. (2020). Football-specific validity of TRACAB's optical video tracking systems. *PLoS ONE, 15*, e0230179. doi:10.1371/journal.pone.0230179.

Lipton, Z. C., Berkowitz, J., & Elkan, C. (2015). A critical review of recurrent neural networks for sequence learning. arXiv preprint arXiv:1506.00019.

Liu, W., Yan, C. C., Liu, J., & Ma, H. (2017). Deep learning based basketball video analysis for intelligent arena application. *Multimedia Tools and Applications, 76*(23), 24983–25001.

Lopes, A. M., & Tenreiro Machado, J. A. (2019). Entropy analysis of soccer dynamics. *Entropy, 21*(2), 187.

Lopez, M. J., & Matthews, G. J. (2015). Building an NCAA men's basketball predictive model and quantifying its success. *Journal of Quantitative Analysis in Sports, 11*(1), 5–12. Retrieved from http://search.ebscohost.com/login.aspx?direct=true&db=s3h&AN=102722690&lang=pt-pt&site=ehost-live&scope=site.

López-Valenciano, A., Ruiz-Pérez, I., Garcia-Gómez, A., Vera-Garcia, F. J., De Ste Croix, M., Myer, G. D., & Ayala, F. (2020). Epidemiology of injuries in professional football: A systematic review and meta-analysis. *British Journal of Sports Medicine, 54*(12), 711–718. doi:10.1136/bjsports-2018–099577.

Lorena, A. C., & de Carvalho, A. C. (2007). Uma introdução às support vector machines. *Revista de Informática Teórica e Aplicada, 14*(2), 43–67.

Lucchesi, M. (2001). *Attacking soccer: A tactical analysis.* Spring City, PA: Reedswain Inc.

Luo, J., Chen, H., Zhang, Q., Xu, Y., Huang, H., & Zhao, X. (2018). An improved grasshopper optimization algorithm with application to financial stress prediction. *Applied Mathematical Modelling, 64*, 654–668. doi:10.1016/j.apm.2018.07.044.

Magill, R., & Anderson, D. (2016). *Motor learning and control: Concepts and applications* (11th ed.). Columbia, NY: McGraw-Hill Education.

Maier, T., Meister, D., Trösch, S., & Wehrlin, J. P. (2018). Predicting biathlon shooting performance using machine learning. *Journal of Sports Sciences, 36*(20), 2333–2339. Retrieved from http://search.ebscohost.com/login.aspx?direct=true&db=s3h&AN=130648934&lang=pt-pt&site=ehost-live&scope=site.

Manning, C. D., Raghavan, P., & Schütze, H. (2008). *Introduction to information retrieval.* Cambridge, UK: Cambridge University Press.

Martínez-Cagigal, V. (2018). *Sample entropy.* Massachusetts: Mathworks.

Martinez-del-Rincon, J., Herrero-Jaraba, E., Raul Gomez, J., Orrite-Urunuela, C., Medrano, C., & Montanes-Laborda, M. A. (2009). Multicamera sport player tracking with Bayesian estimation of measurements. *Optical Engineering, 48*(4). doi:10.1117/1.3114605.

Martins, R. G., Martins, A. S., Neves, L. A., Lima, L. V., Flores, E. L., & do Nascimento, M. Z. (2017). Exploring polynomial classifier to predict match results in football championships. *Expert Systems with Applications, 83*, 79–93. doi:10.1016/j.eswa.2017.04.040.

McCarthy, J. (1997). AI as sport. *Science, 276*(5318), 1518–1519.

McGinley, J. L., Baker, R., Wolfe, R., & Morris, M. E. (2009). The reliability of three-dimensional kinematic gait measurements: A systematic review. *Gait Posture, 29*, 360–359.

McInnes, S. E., Carlson, J. S., Jones C. J., & McKenna, M. J. (1995). The physiological load imposed on basketball players during competition. *Journal of Sport Sciences, 13*, 387–397.

Mello, R. G., Oliveira, L. F., & Nadal, J. (2007). Digital Butterworth filter for subtracting noise from low magnitude surface electromyogram. *Computer Methods and Programs in Biomedicine, 87*(1), 28–35.

Memmert, D., & Perl, J. (2009a). Analysis and simulation of creativity learning by means of artificial neural networks. *Human Movement Science, 28*(2), 263–282. doi:10.1016/j.humov.2008.07.006.

Memmert, D., & Perl, J. (2009b). Game creativity analysis using neural networks. *Journal of Sports Sciences, 27*(2), 139–149. doi:10.1080/02640410802442007.

Menayo, R., Encarnación, A., Gea, G. M., & Marcos, P. J. (2014). Sample entropy-based analysis of differential and traditional training effects on dynamic balance in healthy people. *Journal of Motor Behavior, 46*(2), 73–82.

Merleau-Ponty, M. (1945). *Phénoménologie de la perception.* Paris: Éditions Gailimard.

Merletti, R., & Di Torino, P. (1999). Standards for reporting EMG data. *Journal of Electromyography and Kinesiology, 9*(1), 3–4.

Meskó, B., Hetényi, G., & Győrffy, Z. (2018). Will artificial intelligence solve the human resource crisis in healthcare? *BMC Health Services Research, 18*(1), 545.

Mezyk, E., & Unold, O. (2011). Machine learning approach to model sport training. *Computers in Human Behavior, 27*(5), 1499–1506. doi:10.1016/j.chb.2010.10.014.

Miah, A. (2017). *Sport 2.0: Transforming sports for a digital world.* Cambridge, MA: MIT Press.

Michaels, C. F., & Zaal, F. T. (2002). Catching fly balls. In S. Bennett, K. Davids, G. J. P. Savelsbergh, & J. van der Kamp (Eds.), *Interceptive actions in sport: Information and movement* (pp. 172–183). London, UK: Routledge.

Min, B., Kim, J., Choe, C., Eom, H., & McKay, R. I. (2008). A compound framework for sports results prediction: A football case study. *Knowledge-Based Systems, 21*(7), 551–562. doi:10.1016/j.knosys.2008.03.016.

Mitchell, T. (1997). *Machine learning.* New York, NY: Mcgraw-Hill.

Moher, D., Liberati, A., Tetzlaff, J., & Altman, D. G. (2009). Preferred reporting items for systematic reviews and meta-analyses: The PRISMA statement. *BMJ, 339,* b2535. doi:10.1136/bmj.b2535.

Montoliu, R., Martín-Félez, R., Torres-Sospedra, J., & Martínez-Usó, A. (2015). Team activity recognition in Association Football using a Bag-of-Words-based method. *Human Movement Science, 41,* 165–178. Retrieved from http://search.ebscohost.com/login.aspx?direct=true&db=s3h&AN=102312573&lang=pt-pt&site=ehost-live&scope=site.

Mooney, R., Corley, G., Godfrey, A., Osborough, C., Quinlan, L. R., & ÓLaighin, G. (2015). Application of video-based methods for competitive swimming analysis: A systematic review. *Sports and Exercise Medicine – Open Journal, 1,* 133–150. doi:10.17140/SEMOJ-1-121.

Mooney, R., Quinlan, L. R., Corley, G., Godfrey, A., Osborough, C., & ÓLaighin, G. (2017). Evaluation of the Finis Swimsense® and the Garmin SwimTM activity monitors for swimming performance and stroke kinematics analysis. *PLoS ONE, 12*(2), e0170902. doi:10.1371/journal.pone.0170902.

Mora, S. V., & Knottenbelt, W. J. (2017). Deep learning for domain-specific action recognition in tennis. In *2017 IEEE Conference on Computer Vision and Pattern Recognition Workshops (CVPRW)* (pp. 170–178). Honolulu, HI: IEEE.

Mortensen, J., & Bornn, L. (2020). Estimating locomotor demands during team play from broadcast-derived tracking data. arXiv:2001.07692. Retrieved from https://arxiv.org/abs/2001.07692.

Motoi, S., Misu, T., Nakada, Y., Yazaki, T., Kobayashi, G., Matsumoto, T., & Yagi, N. (2012). Bayesian event detection for sport games with hidden Markov model. *Pattern Analysis and Applications, 15*(1), 59–72. doi:10.1007/s10044-011-0238-6.

Moura, F. A., Martins, L. E. B., Anido, R. D. O., De Barros, R. M. L., & Cunha, S. A. (2012). Quantitative analysis of Brazilian football players' organisation on the pitch. *Sports Biomechanics, 11*(1), 85–96.

Muazu Musa, R., P. P. Abdul Majeed, A., Taha, Z., Chang, S. W., Ab. Nasir, A. F., & Abdullah, M. R. (2019). A machine learning approach of predicting high potential archers by means of physical fitness indicators. *Plos ONE, 14*(1), e0209638. doi:10.1371/journal.pone.0209638.

Mündermann, L., Corazza, S., & Andriacchi, T. P. (2006). The evolution of methods for the capture of human movement leading to markerless motion capture for biomechanical applications. *Journal of NeuroEngineering and Rehabilitation, 3*, 6. doi:10.1186/1743-0003-3-6.

Najafabadi, M. M., Villanustre, F., Khoshgoftaar, T. M., Seliya, N., Wald, R., & Muharemagic, E. (2015). Deep learning applications and challenges in big data analytics. *Journal of Big Data, 2*(1), 1.

Nakano, N., Sakura, T., Ueda, K., Omura, L., Kimura, A., Iino, Y., Fukashiro, S., & Yoshioka, S. (2020). Evaluation of 3D markerless motion capture accuracy using openpose with multiple video cameras. *Frontiers in Sports and Active Living, 2*, 50. doi:10.3389/fspor.2020.00050.

Nargesian, F., Samulowitz, H., Khurana, U., Khalil, E. B., & Turaga, D. S. (2017). Learning feature engineering for classification. In *Proceedings of the Twenty-Sixth International Joint Conference on Artificial Intelligence (IJCAI)* (pp. 2529–2535). Melbourne, Australia: IJCAI.

Navarro, I., & Matía, F. (2009). A proposal of a set of metrics for collective movement of robots. In *Online Proceedings of Robotics: Science and Systems Workshop on Good Experimental Methodology in Robotics*. Seattle, WA: The MIT Press.

Nayel, H. A., & Shashrekha, H. L. (2019). Integrating dictionary feature into a deep learning model for disease named entity recognition. arXiv:1911.01600.

Nemec, B., Petric, T., Babic, J., & Supej, M. (2014). Estimation of alpine skier posture using machine learning techniques. *Sensors, 14*(10), 18898–18914. doi:10.3390/s141018898.

Nilsson, N. J. (2014). *Principles of artificial intelligence*. Burlington, MA: Morgan Kaufmann.

Nüesch, C., Roos, E., Pagenstert, G., & Mündermann, A. (2017). Measuring joint kinematics of treadmill walking and running: Comparison between an inertial sensor based system and a camera-based system. *Journal of Biomechanics, 57*, 32–38. doi:10.1016/j.jbiomech.2017.03.015.

Nunome, H., Ikegami, Y., Kozakai, R., Apriantono, T., & Sano, S. (2006a). Segmental dynamics of soccer instep kicking with the preferred and non-preferred leg. *Journal of Sports Sciences, 24*(5), 529–541.

Nunome, H., Lake, M., Georgakis, A., & Stergioulas, L. K. (2006b). Impact phase kinematics of instep kicking in soccer. *Journal of Sports Sciences, 24*(1), 11–22.

Ofoghi, B., Zeleznikow, J., MacMahon, C., & Dwyer, D. (2013). Supporting athlete selection and strategic planning in track cycling omnium: A statistical and machine learning approach. *Information Sciences, 233*, 200–213. doi:10.1016/j.ins.2012.12.050.

Ofoghi, B., Zeleznikow, J., MacMahon, C., & Raab, M. (2013). Data mining in elite sports: A review and a framework. *Measurement in Physical Education and Exercise Science, 17*(3), 171–186. doi:10.1080/1091367X.2013.805137.

Omodei, M., & McLennan, J. (1994). Studying complex decision making in natural settings: Using a head-mounted video camera to study competitive orienteering. *Perceptual and Motor Skills, 79*, 1411–1425. doi:10.2466/pms.1994.79.3f.1411.

Orth, D., Davids, K., Chow, J. Y., & Brymer, E., & Seifert, L. (2018a). Behavioural repertoire influences the rate and nature of learning in climbing: Implications for individualised learning design in preparation for extreme sports participation. *Frontiers in Psychology, 9*, 949. doi:10.3389/fpsyg.2018.00949.

Orth, D., Davids, K., & Seifert, L. (2018b). Constraints representing a meta-stable régime facilitate exploration during practice and transfer of learning in a complex multi-articular task. *Human Movement Science, 57*, 291–302. doi:10.1016/j.humov.2017.09.007.

Orth, D., Kerr, G., Davids, K., & Seifert, L. (2017). Analysis of relations between spatiotemporal movement regulation and performance of discrete actions reveals functionality in skilled climbing. *Frontiers in Psychology, 8*, 1744. doi:10.3389/fpsyg.2017.01744.

Osgnach, C., Poser, S., Bernardini, R., Rinaldo, R., & Di Prampero, P. E. (2010). Energy cost and metabolic power in elite soccer: A new match analysis approach. *Medicine & Science in Sports & Exercise, 42*(1), 170–178.

Oswald, F. (2020). Future research directions for big data in psychology. In S. Woo, L. Tay, & R. Proctor (Eds.), *Big data in psychological research* (pp. 427–442). Washington, DC: American Psychological Association.

Owramipur, F., Eskandarian, P., & Mozneb, F. S. (2013). Football result prediction with Bayesian network in Spanish League-Barcelona team. *International Journal of Computer Theory and Engineering, 5*(5), 812.

Panjan, A., Šarabon, N., & Filipčič, A. (2010). Prediction of the successfulness of tennis players with machine learning methods. Predvidanje natjecateljske uspješnosti tenisača korištenjem metoda strojnog učenja. *Kinesiology, 42*(1), 98–106. Retrieved from http://search.ebscohost.com/login.aspx?direct=true&db=s3h&AN=52950514&lang=pt-pt&site=ehost-live&scope=site.

Pappalardo, L., & Cintia, P. (2018). Quantifying the relation between performance and success in soccer. *Advances in Complex Systems, 21*(3–4). doi:10.1142/s021952591750014x.

Pappalardo, L., Cintia, P., Ferragina, P., Massucco, E., Pedreschi, D., & Giannotti, F. (2019). PlayeRank: Data-driven performance evaluation and player ranking in soccer via a machine learning approach. *ACM Transactions on Intelligent Systems and Technology, 10*(5). doi:10.1145/3343172.

Passos, P., Araújo, D., Davids, K., Gouveia, L., Milho, J., & Serpa, S. (2008). Information-governing dynamics of attacker-defender interactions in youth rugby union. *Journal of Sports Sciences, 26*(13), 1421–1429. doi:10.1080/02640410802208986.

Passos, P., Araújo, D., Davids, K., Gouveia, L., & Serpa, S. (2006). Interpersonal dynamics in sport: The role of artificial neural networks and 3-D analysis. *Behavior Research Methods, 38*(4), 683–691. doi:10.3758/bf03193901.

Passos, P., Araújo, D., Davids, K., Gouveia, L., Serpa, S., Milho, J., & Fonseca, S. (2009). Interpersonal pattern dynamics and adaptive behavior in multi-agent neurobiological systems: A conceptual model and data. *Journal of Motor Behavior, 41*, 445–459.

Passos, P., Araújo, D., & Volossovitch, A. (2017). *Performance analysis in team sports*. London, UK: Routledge.

Passos, P., Davids, K., Araújo, D., Paz, N., Minguéns, J., & Mendes, J. (2011). Networks as a novel tool for studying team ball sports as complex social systems. *Journal of Science and Medicine in Sport, 14*(2), 170–176.

Pavlakos, G., Zhou, X., & Daniilidis, K. (2018). Ordinal depth supervision for 3D human pose estimation. *Proceedings of the IEEE conference on computer vision and pattern recognition* (pp. 7307–7316). doi:10.1109/CVPR.20 18.00763.

Pavllo, D., Feichtenhofer, C., Grangier, D., & Auli, M. (2019). 3D human pose estimation in video with temporal convolutions and semi-supervised training. *Proceedings of the IEEE conference on computer vision and pattern recognition* (pp. 7753–7762). doi:10.1109/CVPR.2019.00794.

Pelz, D. (2000). *Putting Bible: The complete guide to mastering the green.* New York, NY: Publication Doubleday.

Pers, J., Bon, M., Kovacic, S., Sibila, M., & Dezman, B. (2002). Observation and analysis of large-scale human motion. *Human Movement Science, 21,* 295–311.

Pfister, A., West, A. M., Bronner, S., & Noah, J. A. (2014). Comparative abilities of Microsoft Kinect and Vicon 3D motion capture for gait analysis. *Journal of Medical Engineering & Technology, 38,* 274–280. doi:10.3109/03091902.2014.909540.

Pinder, R. A., Davids, K., Renshaw, I., Araújo, D. (2011a). Representative learning design and functionality of research and practice in sport. *Journal of Sport & Exercise Psychology, 33,* 146–155.

Pinder, R. A., Davids, K., Renshaw, I. & Araújo, D. (2011b). Manipulating informational constraints shapes movement re-organisation in interceptive actions. *Attention, Perception, & Psychophysics, 73,* 1242–1254.

Pobiruchin, M., Suleder, J., Zowalla, R., & Wiesner, M. (2017). Accuracy and adoption of wearable technology used by active citizens: A marathon event field study. *JMIR mHealth and uHealth, 5*(2), e24. doi:10.2196/mhealth.6395.

Poitras, I., Dupuis, F., Bielmann, M., Campeau-Lecours, A., Mercier, C., Bouyer, L. J., & Roy, J.-S. (2019). Validity and reliability of wearable sensors for joint angle estimation: A systematic review. *Sensors, 19*(7), 1–17. doi:10.3390/s19071555.

Polikar, R. (2012). Ensemble learning. In C. Zhang, & Y. Ma (Eds.). *Ensemble machine learning* (pp. 1–34). Boston, MA: Springer.

Priddy, K. L. (2005). *Artificial neural networks: An introduction* (Vol. 68). Washington, DC: SPIE Press.

Proakis, J. G., & Manolakis, D. G. (1996). *Digital signal processing. Principles, algorithms, and applications.* Upper Saddle River, NJ: Prentice Hall.

Proctor, R., & Xiong, A. (2020). From small-scale experiments to big data: Challenges and opportunities for experimental psychologists. In S. Woo, L. Tay, & R. Proctor (Eds.), *Big data in psychological research* (pp. 35–58). Washington, DC: American Psychological Association.

Psycharakis, S. G., & Sanders, R. H. (2008). Shoulder and hip roll changes during 200-m front crawl swimming. *Medicine & Science in Sports & Exercise, 40*(12), 2129–2136. doi:10.1249/MSS.0b013e31818160bc.

Raedeke, T. D., & Smith, A. L. (2001). Development and preliminary validation of an athlete burnout measure. *Journal of Sport and Exercise Psychology, 23*(4), 281–306.

Ram, N., & Diehl, M. (2015). Multiple time-scale design and analysis: Pushing towards realtime modeling of complex developmental processes. In M. Diehl, K. Hooker, & M. Sliwinski (Eds.), *Handbook of intraindividual variability across the lifespan* (pp. 308–323). New York, NY: Routledge.

Ramos, J., Lopes, R. J., Marques, P., & Araújo, D. (2017). Hypernetworks reveal compound variables that capture cooperative and competitive interactions in a soccer match. *Frontiers in Psychology, 8,* 1379. doi:10.3389/fpsyg.2017.01379.

Ramos, J. P., Lopes, R. J., & Araújo, D. (2020). Interactions between soccer teams reveal both design and emergence: Cooperation, competition and Zipf-Mandelbrot regularity. *Chaos, Solitons & Fractals, 137,* 109872. doi:10.1016/j.chaos.2020.109872.

Randers, M., Mujikab, I., Hewitt, A., Santisteban, J., Bischoff, R., Solano, R., Zubillaga, A., Peltola, E., Krustrup, P., & Mohr, M. (2010). Application of four different football match analysis systems: A comparative study. *Journal of Sports Sciences, 28*(2), 171–182. doi:10.1080/02640410903428525.

Ravasz, E., & Barabási, A. L. (2003). Hierarchical organization in complex networks. *Physical Review E, 67*(2), 026122. doi:10.1103/PhysRevE.67.026112.

Razali, N., Mustapha, A., Yatim, F. A., & Ab Aziz, R. (2017). Predicting football matches results using Bayesian networks for English Premier League (EPL). *IOP Conference Series: Materials Science and Engineering, 226*(1), 012099.

Reed, E. S. (1993). The intention to use a specific affordance: A conceptual framework for psychology. In R. H. Wozniak & K. W. Fischer (Eds.), *Development in context: Acting and thinking in specific environments* (pp. 45–76). Hillsdale, NJ: Erlbaum.

Rein, R. (2012). Measurement methods to analyze changes in coordination during motor learning from a non-linear perspective. *The Open Sports Sciences Journal, 5*(1), 36–48. doi:10.2174/1875399X01205010036.

Rein, R., Button, C., Davids, K., & Summers, J. (2010). Cluster analysis of movement pattern dynamics in multi-articular actions. *Motor Control, 14*, 211–239.

Rein, R., & Memmert, D. (2016). Big data and tactical analysis in elite soccer: Future challenges and opportunities for sports science. *Springerplus, 5*, 1410.

Renshaw, I., Davids, K., Araújo, D., Lucas, A., Roberts, W. M., Newcombe, D. J., & Franks B. (2019). Evaluating weaknesses of "perceptual-cognitive training" and "brain training" methods in sport: An ecological dynamics critique. *Frontiers in Psychology, 9*, 2468. doi:10.3389/fpsyg.2018.02468.

Reynolds, D. A. (2009). Gaussian mixture models. In S. Z. Li, & A. Jain (Eds.), *Encyclopedia of Biometric* (p. 741). Boston, MA: Springer.

Ribeiro, J., Davids, K., Araújo, D., Silva, P., Ramos, J., Lopes, R., & Garganta. J. (2019). The role of hypernetworks as a multilevel methodology for modelling and understanding dynamics of team sports performance. *Sports Medicine, 49*(9), 1337–1344. doi:10.1007/s40279-019-01104-x.

Ribeiro, J., Figueiredo, P., Morais, S., Alves, F., Toussaint, H., Vilas-Boas, J. P., & Fernandes, R. J. (2017). Biomechanics, energetics and coordination during extreme swimming intensity: Effect of performance level. *Journal of Sports Sciences, 35*(16), 1614–1621. doi:10.1080/02640414.2016.1227079.

Rich, E. (1983). *Artificial intelligence.* New York, NY: McGraw-Hill.

Richman, J. S., & Moorman, J. R. (2000). Physiological time-series analysis using approximate entropy and sample entropy. *American Journal of Physiology-Heart and Circulatory Physiology, 278*(6), H2039–H2049.

Rietveld, E., Denys, D., & Van Westen, M. (2018). Ecological-enactive cognition as engaging with a rich landscape of affordances: The skilled intentionality framework (SIF). In A. Newen, L. De Bruin, & S. Gallagher (Eds.), *The Oxford handbook of 4E cognition.* New York, NY: Oxford University Press.

Rindal, O. M. H., Seeberg, T. M., Tjonnas, J., Haugnes, P., & Sandbakk, O. (2018). Automatic classification of sub-techniques in classical cross-country skiing using a machine learning algorithm on micro-sensor data. *Sensors, 18*(1). doi:10.3390/s18010075.

Rish, I. (2001). An empirical study of the naive Bayes classifier. *IJCAI 2001 workshop on empirical methods in artificial intelligence, 3*(22), 41–46.

Roberts, S., Trewartha, G., & Stokes, K. (2006). A comparison of time–motion analysis methods for field-based sports. *International Journal of Sports Physiology and Performance, 1*, 388–399.

Robertson, S., Spencer, B., Back, N., & Farrow, D. (2019). A rule induction framework for the determination of representative learning design in skilled performance. *Journal of Sports Sciences, 37*(11), 1280–1285. doi:10.1080/02640414.2018.1555905.

Robinson, A. C. (2011). Highlighting in geovisualization. *Cartography and Geographic Information Science, 38*, 373–383.

Rodrigues, A. C. N., Pereira, A. S., Mendes, R. M. S., Araújo, A. G., Couceiro, M. S., & Figueiredo, A. J. (2020). Using artificial intelligence for pattern recognition in a sports context. *Sensors, 20*(11), 3040.

Ross, G. B., Dowling, B., Troje, N. F., Fischer, S. L., & Graham, R. B. (2018). Objectively differentiating movement patterns between elite and novice athletes. *Medicine and Science in Sports and Exercise, 50*(7), 1457–1464. doi:10.1249/mss.0000000000001571.

Rossi, A., Pappalardo, L., Cintia, P., Iaia, F. M., Fernandez, J., & Medina, D. (2018). Effective injury forecasting in soccer with GPS training data and machine learning. *Plos ONE, 13*(7). doi:10.1371/journal.pone.0201264.

Rothwell, M., Davids, K., Stone, J., Araújo, D., & Shuttleworth, R. (2020). The talent development process as enhancing athlete functionality: Creating forms of life in an ecological niche. In J. Baker, S. Cobley, J. Schorer, & N. Wattie (Eds.), *Routledge handbook of talent identification and development in sport* (2nd Ed.). Abingdon, UK: Routledge.

Ruddy, J. D., Shield, A. J., Maniar, N., Williams, M. D., Duhig, S., Timmins, R. G., Hickey, J., Bourne, M. N., & Opar, D. A. (2018). Predictive modeling of hamstring strain injuries in elite australian footballers. *Medicine and Science in Sports and Exercise, 50*(5), 906–914. doi:10.1249/mss.0000000000001527.

Russell, S., & Norvig, P. (2002). *Artificial intelligence: A modern approach*. Essex, England: Pearson Education Limited.

Russell, S., & Norvig, P. (Eds.). (2003). Constraint satisfaction problems. In *Artificial Intelligence: A Modern Approach* (pp. 137–160). Essex, England: Pearson Education Limited.

Sabatini, A. M. (2011). Estimating three-dimensional orientation of human body parts by inertial/magnetic sensing. *Sensors, 11*(2), 1489–1525. doi:10.3390/s110201489.

Sadeghizadeh, M. R., Saranjam, B., & Kamali, R. (2017). Experimental and numerical investigation of high speed swimmer motion drag force in different depths from free surface. *Journal of Applied Fluid Mechanics, 10*(1), 343–352.

Safavian, S. R., & Landgrebe, D. (1991). A survey of decision tree classifier methodology. *IEEE transactions on systems, man, and cybernetics, 21*(3), 660–674.

Sak, H., Senior, A., & Beaufays, F. (2014). Long short-term memory recurrent neural network architectures for large scale acoustic modeling. In *Fifteenth Annual Conference of the International Speech Communication Association* (pp. 338–342). Singapore: ISCA.

Samuel, A. L. (1959). Some studies in machine learning using the game of checkers. *IBM Journal of Research and Development, 3*(3), 210–229. doi:10.1147/rd.33.0210.

Sanchez-Algarra, P., & Anguera, M. T. (2013). Qualitative/quantitative integration in the inductive observational study of interactive behaviour: Impact of recording and coding predominating perspectives. *Quality y Quantity, 47*(2), 1237–1257. doi: 10.1007/s11135-012-9764-6.

Sandau, M., Koblauch, H., Moeslund, T. B., Aanæs, H., Alkjær, T., & Simonsen, E. B. (2014). Markerless motion capture can provide reliable 3D gait kinematics in the sagittal and frontal plane. *Medical Engineering & Physics, 36*(9), 1168–1175. doi:10.1016/j.medengphy.2014.07.007.

Sandnes, F. E., & Jian, H.-L. (2004). Pair-wise varibility index: Evaluating the cognitive difficulty of using mobile text entry systems. In S. Brewster & M. Dunlop (Eds.), *Mobile human–computer interaction* (pp. 347–350). Heidelberg, Germany: Springer.

Sarmento, H., Bradley, P., Anguera, M. T., Polido, T., Resende, R., & Campaniço, J. (2016). Quantifying the offensive sequences that result in goals in elite futsal matches. *Journal of Sports Sciences, 34*(7), 621–629. doi:10.1080/02640414.2015.106 6024.

Schlipsing, M., Salmen, J., Tschentscher, M., & Igel, C. (2017). Adaptive pattern recognition in real-time video-based soccer analysis. *Journal of Real-Time Image Processing, 13*(2), 345–361. doi:10.1007/s11554-014-0406-1.

Schmidt, A. (2012). Movement pattern recognition in basketball free-throw shooting. *Human Movement Science, 31*(2), 360–382. doi:10.1016/j.humov.2011.01.003.

Schmitz, A., Ye, M., Shapiro, R., Yang, R., & Noehren, B. (2014). Accuracy and repeatability of joint angles measured using a single camera markerless motion capture system. *Journal of Biomechanics, 47*, 587–591. doi:10.1016/j.jbiomech.2013.11.031.

Schölkopf, B. (2001). The kernel trick for distances. In T. K. Leen, T. G. Dietterich & V. Tresp (Eds.), *Advances in neural information processing systems* (pp. 301–307). Massachusetts: Massachusetts Institute of Technology Press.

Schulte, O., Khademi, M., Gholami, S., Zhao, Z., Javan, M., & Desaulniers, P. (2017). A Markov Game model for valuing actions, locations, and team performance in ice hockey. *Data Mining and Knowledge Discovery, 31*(6), 1735–1757. doi:10.1007/ s10618-017-0496-z.

Schuster, M., & Paliwal, K. K. (1997). Bidirectional recurrent neural networks. *IEEE Transactions on Signal Processing, 45*(11), 2673–2681.

Schwartz, B. (2004). *The paradox of choice: Why more is less.* New York, NY: HarperCollins Publishers.

Scott, M. T. U., Scott, T. J., & Kelly, V. G. (2016). The validity and reliability of global positioning systems in team sport: A brief review. *Journal of Strength and Conditioning Research, 30*(5), 1470–1490. doi:10.1519/JSC.0000000000001221.

Seel, T., Raisch, J., & Schauer, T. (2014). IMU-based joint angle measurement for gait analysis. *Sensors, 14*(4), 6891–6909. doi:10.3390/s140406891.

Seifert, L., Boulanger, J., Orth, D., & Davids, K. (2015). Environmental design shapes perceptual-motor exploration, learning and transfer in climbing. *Frontiers in Psychology, 6*, 1819. doi:10.3389/fpsyg.2015.01819.

Seifert, L., Button, C., & Davids, K. (2013). Key properties of expert movement systems in sport: An ecological dynamics perspective. *Sport Medicine, 43*(1), 167–178.

Seifert, L., & Davids, K. (2012). Intentions, perceptions and actions constrain functional intra- and inter-individual variability in the acquisition of expertise in individual sports. *Open Journal of Sport Sciences, 5*, 68–75.

Seifert, L., Hacques, G., Rivet, R., & Legreneur, P. (2020). Assessment of fluency dynamics in climbing. *Sport Biomechanics.* doi:10.1080/14763141.2020.1830161.

Seifert, L., Komar, J., Barbosa, T., Toussaint, H. M., Millet, G., & Davids, K. (2014). Coordination pattern variability provides functional adaptations to constraints in swimming performance. *Sports Medicine, 44*(10), 1333–1345.

Seifert, L., Komar, J., Hérault, R., & Chollet, D. (2014). Using inertial measurement unit for coordination pattern detection and recognition in breaststroke. In B. Mason (Ed.), *XIIth International Symposium for Biomechanics and Medicine in Swimming XII* (pp. 235–242). Canberra, Australia: Australian Institute of Sport.

Seifert, L., Orth, D., Boulanger, J., Dovgalecs, V., Hérault, R., & Davids K. (2014). Climbing skill and complexity of climbing wall design: Assessment of jerk as a novel indicator of performance fluency. *Journal of Applied Biomechanics, 30*(5), 619–625.

Seifert, L., Orth, D., Mantel, B., Boulanger, J., Hérault, R., & Dicks, M. (2018). Affordance realisation in climbing: Learning and transfer. *Frontiers in Psychology, 9*, 820. doi:10.3389/fpsyg.2018.00820.

Seifert, L., Schnitzler, C., Aujouannet, Y., Carter, M., Rouard, A., & Chollet, D. (2006). Comparison of subjective and objective methods of determination of stroke phases to analyse arm coordination in front-crawl. *Portuguese Journal of Sport Sciences, 6*(Supl. 2), 92–94.

Shan, G., & Westerhoff, P. (2005). Soccer: Full-body kinematic characteristics of the maximal instep soccer kick by male soccer players and parameters related to kick quality. *Sports Biomechanics, 4*(1), 59–72.

Sibella, F., Frosio, I., Schena, F., & Borghese, N. A. (2007). 3D analysis of the body center of mass in rock climbing. *Human Movement Science, 26*(6), 841–852. doi:10.1016/j.humov.2007.05.008.

Sillanpää, V., & Heino, O. (2013). *Forecasting football match results – A study on modeling principles and efficiency of fixed-odds betting markets in football.* (Master's thesis on Quantitative Methods of Economics). Department of Information and Service Economy. Aalto University, School of Business.

Silvatti, A. P., Cerveri, P., Telles, T., Dias, F. A. S., Baroni, G., & Barros, R. M. L. (2013). Quantitative underwater 3D motion analysis using submerged video cameras: Accuracy analysis and trajectory reconstruction. *Computer Methods in Biomechanics and Biomedical Engineering, 16*, 1240–1248. doi:10.1080/10255842.2012.664637.

Simbaña-Escobar, D., Hellard, P., Pyne, D., & Seifert, L. (2018a). Functional role of movement and performance variability: Adaptation of front crawl swimmers to competitive swimming constraints. *Journal of Applied Biomechanics, 34*(1), 53–64. doi:10.1123/jab.2017–0022.

Simbaña-Escobar, D., Hellard, P., & Seifert L. (2018b). Modelling stroking parameters in competitive sprint swimming: Understanding inter- and intra-lap variability to assess pacing management. *Human Movement Science, 61*, 219–230.

Sinar, E. F. (2015). Data visualization. In S. Tonidandel, E. B. King, & J. M. Cortina (Eds.), *Big data at work: The data science revolution and organizational psychology* (pp. 129–171). New York, NY: Routledge.

SkillCorner. (2020). A new world of performance insight from video tracking technology. Retrieved from https://medium.com/skillcorner/a-new-world-of-performance-insight-from-video-tracking-technology-f0d7c0deb767.

Sokolova, M., Japkowicz, N., & Szpakowicz, S. (2006). Beyond accuracy, F-score and ROC: A family of discriminant measures for performance evaluation. In Sattar, A. & Kang, B. (Eds.), *Australasian joint conference on artificial intelligence* (pp. 1015–1021). Berlin, Heidelberg: Springer.

Song, Q., Liu, M., Tang, C., & Long, L. (2020). Applying principles of big data to the workplace and talent analytics. In S. Woo, L. Tay, & R. Proctor (Eds.), *Big data in psychological research* (pp. 319–344). Washington, DC: American Psychological Association.

Spann, M., & Skiera, B. (2009). Sports forecasting: A comparison of the forecast accuracy of prediction markets, betting odds and tipsters. *Journal of Forecasting, 28*(1), 55–72.

Stepp, N., & Turvey, M. T. (2010). On strong anticipation. *Cognitive Systems Research*, *11*, 148–164.

Stone, J., Strafford, B. W., North, J. S., Toner, C., & Davids, K. (2018). Effectiveness and efficiency of virtual reality designs to enhance athlete development: An ecological dynamics perspective. *Movement and Sport Science/Science et Motricité*, *102*, 51–60. doi:10.1051/sm/2018031.

Stone, K. J., & Oliver, J. L. (2009). The effect of 45 minutes of soccer-specific exercise on the performance of soccer skills. *International Journal of Sports Physiology and Performance*, *4*(2), 163–175.

Takahashi, M., Yokozawa, S., Mitsumine, H., & Mishina, T. (2018). Real-time ball-position measurement using multi-view cameras for live football broadcast. *Multimedia Tools and Applications*, *77*(18), 23729–23750. doi:10.1007/s11042-018-5694-1.

Tang, B., Kay, S., & He, H. (2016). Toward optimal feature selection in naive Bayes for text categorization. *IEEE Transactions on Knowledge and Data Engineering*, *28*(9), 2508–2521.

Tavana, M., Azizi, F., Azizi, F., & Behzadian, M. (2013). A fuzzy inference system with application to player selection and team formation in multi-player sports. *Sport Management Review*, *16*(1), 97–110.

Tay, L., Jebb, A. T., & Woo, S. E. (2017). Video capture of human behaviors: Toward a big data approach. *Current Opinion in Behavioral Sciences*, *18*, 17–22.

Taylor, L., Miller, E., & Kaufman, K. R. (2017). Static and dynamic validation of inertial measurement units. *Gait & Posture*, *57*, 80–84. doi:10.1016/j.gaitpost.2017.05.026.

Teufl, W., Miezal, M., Taetz, B., Fröhlich, M., & Bleser, G. (2018). Validity, test-retest reliability and long-term stability of magnetometer free inertial sensor based 3D joint kinematics. *Sensors*, *18*(1980), 1–22. doi:10.3390/s18071980.

Thewlis, D., Bishop, C., Daniell, N., & Paul, G. (2013). Next-generation low-cost motion capture systems can provide comparable spatial accuracy to high-end systems. *Journal of Applied Biomechanics*, *29*(1), 112–117. doi:10.1123/jab.29.1.112.

Trapattoni, G. (2000). *Coaching high performance soccer*. Spring City, PA: Reedswain Inc.

Travassos, B., Araújo, D., Duarte, R., & McGarry, T. (2012). Spatiotemporal coordination behaviors in futsal (indoor football) are guided by informational game constraints. *Human Movement Science*, *31*(4), 932–945. doi:10.1016/j.humov.2011.10.004.

Tsai, W. (2002). Social structure of "coopetition" within a multiunit organization: Coordination, competition, and intraorganizational knowledge sharing. *Organization Science*, *13*(2), 179–190.

Turvey, M. & Carello, C. (1981). Cognition: The view from ecological realism. *Cognition*, *10*, 313–321.

van Den Brink, R., & Borm, P. (2002). Digraph competitions and cooperative games. *Theory and Decision*, *53*(4), 327–342.

Van Winckel, J., Tenney, D., Helsen, W., McMillan, K., Meert, J., & Bradley, P. (2014). *Fitness in soccer – The science and practical aplicattion*. Levene: Moveo Ergo Sum.

Vigotsky, A. D., Halperin, I., Lehman, G. J., Trajano, G. S., & Vieira, T. M. (2018). Interpreting signal amplitudes in surface electromyography studies in sport and rehabilitation sciences. *Frontiers in Physiology*, *8*, 985.

Vilar, L., Araújo, D., Davids, K., & Button, C. (2012). The role of ecological dynamics in analysing performance in team sports. *Sports Medicine*, *42*(1), 1–10. doi:10.2165/11596520-000000000-00000.

Vilar, L., Araújo, D., Davids, K., Travassos, B., Duarte, R., & Parreira, J. (2014). Interpersonal coordination tendencies supporting the creation/prevention of goal scoring opportunities in futsal. *European Journal of Sport Science*, *14*(1), 28–35.

Waldron, M., Worsfold, P., Twist, C., & Lamb, K. (2011). Concurrent validity and test- retest reliability of a global positioning system (GPS) and timing gates to assess sprint performance variables. *Journal of Sports Sciences*, *29*(15), 1613–1619. doi:10.108 0/02640414.2011.608703.

Wallgrün, J. O., Karimzadeh, M., MacEachren, A. M., & Pezanowski, S. (2018). GeoCorpora: Building a corpus to test and train microblog geoparsers. *International Journal of Geographical Information Science*, *32*, 1–29.

Ward, P., Schraagen, J., Gore, J., & Roth, E. (2020). *The oxford handbook of expertise*. Oxford, UK: Oxford University Press.

Watts, D. J. (2002). A simple model of information cascades on random networks. *Proceedings of the National Academy of Science of the U.S.A.*, *99*(9), 5766–5771. doi:10.1073/pnas.082090499.

Watts, P. B., España-Romero, V., Ostrowski, M. L., & Jensen, R. L. (2020). Change in geometric entropy with repeated ascents in rock climbing. *Sports Biomechanics*, *30*, 1–10. doi:10.1080/14763141.2019.1635636.

Whiteside, D., Cant, O., Connolly, M., & Reid, M. (2017). Monitoring hitting load in tennis using inertial sensors and machine learning. *International Journal of Sports Physiology and Performance*, *12*(9), 1212–1217. doi:10.1123/ijspp.2016-0683.

Willmott, A. G. B., James, C. A., Bliss, A., Leftwich, R. A., & Maxwell, N. S. (2019). A comparison of two global positioning system devices for team-sport running protocols. *Journal of Biomechanics*, *23*(83), 324–328. doi:10.1016/j.jbiomech.2018.11.044.

Wilson, D. J., Smith, B. K., Gibson, J. K., Choe, B. K., Gaba, B. C., & Voelz, J. T. (1999). Accuracy of digitization using automated and manual methods. *Physical Therapy*, *79*(6) 558–566.

Withagen, R., Araújo, D., & de Poel, H. J. (2017). Inviting affordances and agency. *New Ideas in Psychology*, *45*, 11–18.

Withagen, R., de Poel, H. J., Araújo, D., & Pepping, G.-J. (2012). Affordances can invite behavior: Reconsidering the relationship between affordances and agency. *New Ideas in Psychology*, *30*, 250–258.

Woo, S., Tay, L., Jebb, A., Ford, M., & Kern, M. (2020). Big Data for enhancing measurement quality. In S. Woo, L. Tay, & R. Proctor (Eds.), *Big data in psychological research* (pp. 59–86). Washington, DC: American Psychological Association.

Woo, S. E., Tay, L., & Proctor, R. W. (Eds.). (2020). *Big data in psychological research*. Washington, DC: American Psychological Association.

Woods, C., McKeown, I., Shuttleworth, R., Davids, K., & Robertson, S. (2019). Training programme designs in professional team sport: An ecological dynamics exemplar. *Human Movement Science*, *66*, 318–326. doi:10.1016/j.humov.2019.05.015.

Wu, M. (2020). wgPlot – Weighted Graph Plot (a better version of gplot). Retrieved from https://www.mathworks.com/matlabcentral/fileexchange/24035-wgplot-weighted-graph-plot-a-better-version-of-gplot. MATLAB Central File Exchange. Accessed April 13, 2020.

Xie, J., Xu, J., Nie, C., & Nie, Q. (2017). Machine learning of swimming data via wisdom of crowd and regression analysis. *Mathematical Biosciences and Engineering*, *14*(2), 511–527. doi:10.3934/mbe.2017031.

Xing, Z., Pei, J., & Keogh, E. (2010). A brief survey on sequence classification. *ACM SIGKDD Explorations Newsletter, 12*(1), 40–48.

Xu, M., Orwell, J., Lowey, L., & Thirde, D. (2005). Architecture and algorithms for tracking football players with multiple cameras. *IEE Proceedings-Vision, Image and Signal Processing, 152*(2), 232–241.

Yadav, J. S., Yadav, M., & Jain, A. (2014). Artificial neural network. *International Journal of Scientific Research and Education, 1*(6), 108–118.

Yeh, H.-P., Stone, J., Churchill, S., Wheat, J., Brymer, E., & Davids, K. (2016). Benefits of green physical activity: An ecological dynamics perspective. *Sports Medicine, 46*, 947–953. doi:10.1007/s40279-015-0374-z.

Yi, Z. (2013). *Convergence analysis of recurrent neural networks* (Vol. 13). Berlin, Germany: Springer Science & Business Media.

Zanone, P. G., & Kelso, J. A. S. (1992). Evolution of behavioural attractors with learning: Nonequilibrium phase transitions. *Journal of Experimental Psychology: Human Perception and Performance, 18*(2), 403–421. doi:10.1037//0096–1523.18.2.403.

Zelic, I., Kononenko, I., Lavrac, N., & Vuga, V. (1997). Diagnosis of sport injuries with machine learning: Explanation of induced decisions. In Kokol, P. Stiglic, B., Brumen, B. & Brest, J. (Eds.), *Proceedings of computer based medical systems* (pp. 195–199). New York, NY: IEEE.

Zhou, H., & Hu, H. (2010). Reducing drifts in the inertial measurements of wrist and elbow positions. *IEEE Transactions on Instrumentation and Measurement, 59*(3), 575–585. doi:10.1109/TIM.2009.2025065.

Zhou, H., Stone, T., Hu, H., & Harris, N. (2008). Use of multiple wearable inertial sensors in upper limb motion tracking. *Medical Engineering & Physics, 30*, 123–133. doi:10.1016/j.medengphy.2006.11.010.

Zhou, Z. H. (2012). *Ensemble methods: Foundations and algorithms.* Boca Raton, FL: CRC Press.

Zimmermann, H. J. (2012). *Fuzzy sets, decision making, and expert systems* (Vol. 10). Dordrecht, Netherlands: Springer Science & Business Media.

INDEX

Printed in the United States
by Baker & Taylor Publisher Services